Workplace Readiness for
HEALTH OCCUPATIONS

Workplace Readiness for
HEALTH OCCUPATIONS

Second Edition

Bruce J. Colbert, M.S., R.R.T.

Associate Professor/Allied Health Director
University of Pittsburgh at Johnstown
Johnstown, Pennsylvania

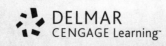
DELMAR
CENGAGE Learning™

Australia • Brazil • Japan • Korea • Mexico • Singapore • Spain • United Kingdom • United States

DELMAR
CENGAGE Learning™

Workplace Readiness for Health Occupations, Second Edition

Bruce J. Colbert

Vice President, Health Care Business Unit: William Brottmiller

Editorial Director: Cathy L. Esperti

Acquisitions Editor: Marah Bellegarde

Developmental Editor: Debra Flis

Editorial Assistant: Jadin Babin-Kavanaugh

Marketing Director: Jennifer McAvey

Marketing Coordinator: Michele Gleason

Production Director: Carolyn Miller

Production Manager: Barbara Bullock

Production Editor: Anne Sherman

For product information and technology assistance, contact us at
Cengage Learning Customer & Sales Support, 1-800-354-9706

For permission to use material from this text or product,
submit all requests online at **www.cengage.com/permissions**
Further permissions questions can be emailed to
permissionrequest@cengage.com

Library of Congress Control Number: 2005014909

ISBN-13: 978-1-4018-7939-6

ISBN-10: 1-4018-7939-X

Delmar
Executive Woods
5 Maxwell Drive
Clifton Park, NY 12065
USA

Cengage Learning is a leading provider of customized learning solutions with office locations around the globe, including Singapore, the United Kingdom, Australia, Mexico, Brazil, and Japan. Locate your local office at:
international.cengage.com/region

Cengage Learning products are represented in Canada by Nelson Education, Ltd.

For your lifelong learning solutions, visit **delmar.cengage.com**

Visit our corporate website at **www.cengage.com**

Notice to the Reader

Printed in U.S.A.

8 9 10 X X X 13 12 11

This book is dedicated to Pap and Gram Cus;
their love, wisdom, and dedication to education
and family have left a legacy that will last
for generations to come.

CONTENTS

Preface / ix

Acknowledgments / xi

About the Author / xii

Introduction / xiii

Developing Portfolios / xv

SECTION ONE
Communicating with Yourself:
Achieving Personal Excellence

CHAPTER 1

Study Skills: Laying the
Foundation 2

Daily Preparation / 3
Pick a Good Time and Place of Study / 4
Use Good Study Habits / 4
Understand the Learning and
    Testing Process / 5
Take Care of Yourself / 7

CHAPTER 2

Personal and Professional
Characteristics for Success 15

Self-Esteem / 17
Self-Confident Attitude / 19
What Is a Professional Attitude? / 20
Trustworthy Attitude / 20
Caring Attitude / 22

Competent Attitude / 23
Positive and Negative Attitudes / 26
Characteristics of Positive Attitudes / 27
Negative Attitudes / 29
Victim Attitude / 29
Changing Negative Attitudes into
    Positive Attitudes / 30
You Can Make a Difference / 30

CHAPTER 3

Setting Goals and
Time Management 42

Setting Goals / 44
Objectives / 46
Types of Goals / 46
Time Management / 49
Using Time Management Techniques / 50
Words to the Wise / 55

CHAPTER 4

Stress Management 67

Understanding Stress / 69
Types of Stress and Its Effects / 70
A Simplified Stress Management System / 73

CHAPTER 5

Thinking and Reasoning Skills 89

Types of Thinking / 90
Critical and Creative Thinking / 92
Directed and Undirected Thinking / 94
The Total Thinking Process / 95

SECTION TWO
Communicating with Others:
Achieving Professional
Excellence

CHAPTER 6

Types of Communication 114

The Communication Process / 115
Types of Communication / 119
Verbal Communication / 122
Written Communication / 124

CHAPTER 7

Communication in Action 135

Barriers to Communication / 136
Listening / 140
Customer Relations / 144
Telephone Etiquette / 145
Technological Communication / 147
Public Speaking / 148
Patient Communication and Education / 149
Recording and Reporting Information / 149

CHAPTER 8

Communication Within an
Organization 156

Communication Networks / 157
Directions of Communication Flow / 159
The Lines of Authority and Responsibility / 160
Working within a Group / 161
Effective Group Participation / 165
Brainstorming / 167
Communication and Meetings / 168

CHAPTER 9

Patient Interaction and
Communication 176

Preparing for the Patient Encounter / 177
The Actual Patient Encounter / 179
Respecting a Patient's Space / 185
Territoriality / 188
You Can Make a Difference / 189

CHAPTER 10

Your First Job as a
Health Care Professional 196

Choosing the Right Position / 197
Preparing a Résumé / 199
Making Contacts and Finding Openings / 201
Writing Cover Letters / 202
The Interview / 204
Your First Job: First and Lasting Impressions / 206
The Importance of Professional Image / 210

CHAPTER 11

Selected Topics 216

Medical Ethics / 217
Euthanasia / 223
Legal Issues / 224
The Patient Care Partnership / 227
Right to Die Issues / 230

Glossary / 241

Index / 245

PREFACE

The major goal of this combined text and workbook is to provide students with a foundation that will ensure their success in health care careers and as lifelong learners.

We all know that health care is one of the fastest growing industries due to an aging population and dramatic technological advances. The face of health care is changing rapidly. The changing environment is due to many factors such as pressures for health care reform, a diverse population, remodeled delivery systems, and so on. However, what will never change is the need for highly trained professional health care providers.

In recognition of this fact, the United States Department of Education funded the National Health Care Skill Standards Project (NHCSSP). This was a highly collaborative and extensive effort among health care workers and administrators, labor leaders, and the education community to define what knowledge and skills are needed to be successful future health care practitioners.

Quoting from this Department of Education report, "These standards serve as a model for education programs and are compatible to other major federal initiatives such as Goals 2000: Educate America Act, the School-to-Work Opportunities Act, and the Carl D. Perkins Vocational Education Act." In addition, it incorporates the 1991 report of the U.S. Secretary of Labor's Commission on Achieving Necessary Skills (SCANS).

The SCANS project set standards for success that individuals need in the modern workplace. The SCANS message to schools is "to look beyond the traditional schoolhouse to roles students will play as workers, citizens, parents etc." Its message to teachers is look beyond your discipline and classroom and connect what the students learn to the outside community.

The author hopes to use the collective wisdom and results of these reports to produce a worktext to give students clear direction and assistance in setting and achieving goals toward successful careers in the health professions. In addition, it will give them "life skills" that will help them reach their full potential.

CHANGES TO THE SECOND EDITION

I am gratified that this nontraditional textbook has been successful enough to warrant a second edition. Health care schools have come to fully realize the importance of focusing on "Workplace Readiness" skills not only for their students' employment success but also for the enhancement of reputation and marketability the school receives from producing students proficient in these areas. In this second edition, I have maintained the "easy to read and relate to" writing style that helps to personally connect the material to the individual student's life experience. While easy to read, the text still challenges students to think and apply information for their personal and professional enhancement. The following list represents "What's New" in this second edition:

- Updated information in the rapidly changing health care areas
- New information that is more clinically applicable such as HIPAA regulations and computerized documentation
- Extension of the critical thinking and application exercises to include case studies to increase integrative and relevant learning
- Internet activities to encourage research and sharing of information beyond the text material
- New sections and discussion on technological communication, communication within meetings, and multiculturalism

I truly hope this project and the enhancements made to the second edition assist health care students in fully realizing their potential not just in their chosen career but also in life.

ACKNOWLEDGMENTS

I wish to acknowledge all the special Health Occupation teachers I have met through my interactive lectures and workshops. You truly are a fun and motivated group. In addition, I wish to thank all those at Delmar Publishers who made this innovative project possible. Finally, a special acknowledgment to my wife Patty, my children Joshua and Jeremy, my parents, brothers and sister, and teachers who have all been the greatest influence in my life.

I also wish to acknowledge the instructors who reviewed the manuscript and provided valuable comments. The reviewers include:

Gwen Barnett, BS, MT (ASCP)
Health Science Education
    Instructor
North High School
Evansville, Indiana

Mary Beth Brown, MRC, BA
Annually Contract Faculty
Sinclair Community College
Dayton, Ohio

Roxann DeLaet, RN, MS
Professor
Sinclair Community College
Dayton, Ohio

Vicki Gentzel, BS
Health Careers Recruitment/
    Retention Specialist
Harrisburg Area Community
    College
Harrisburg, Pennsylvania

Tina M. Peer, BSN, RN
Instructor
Registered Nursing and Allied
    Health Programs
College of Southern Idaho
Twin Falls, Idaho

Maggie Thomas, PT, MA
PTA Program Coordinator
Kirkwood Community College
Cedar Rapids, Iowa

Robert W. Wilcosky, MEd, RRT
Professor Emeritus/Advisor
Medical Center Campus
Miami Dade College

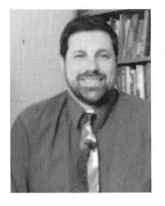

ABOUT THE AUTHOR

Bruce Colbert is a clinical associate professor and director of the Allied Health Department at the University of Pittsburgh at Johnstown. He has authored four books, and has given over 150 invited lectures and workshops at both the regional and national level. Many of his workshops are devoted to stress and time management, enhancing critical and creative thinking, and developing effective decision-making skills. He is an avid basketball player and outdoorsman.

INTRODUCTION

This worktext is not about math or science. It will not ask you to memorize massive amounts of information or complex formulas. This book is about *you*. What do you wish to become, and how do you plan on getting there?

This worktext explores who you are. This should be a hard but worthwhile exploration. Your education can be the ticket to this wondrous and productive journey, but only you can choose the path and determine how hard you are going to work. Sounds corny and you may have heard it all before, but think about it.

Right now you are preparing for the rest of your life. The knowledge and skills you obtain within this worktext can help you achieve your full potential. Section 1 of the worktext focuses on self-communication. This section focuses on *you*. Only you can ensure that you achieve personal and professional excellence. Therefore, the most important personal relationship you must establish is with yourself.

We all know how crucial good communication skills can be in our relationships with others. But what about communication within ourselves? Positive self-communication is the "foundation" upon which to build a successful personal and professional life.

Section 1 will help you determine your strengths and identify areas for improvement. It will assist you in developing action plans and achievable goals to improve your chance of success. It will make you think about who you are and what you wish to become.

Section 2 looks at and improves your communication skills with others. This section discusses communication at an interpersonal level within a group, team, or organization. Basic communication skills are stressed along with their application to success "on the job."

In addition, Section 2 focuses on job-seeking skills. It emphasizes that the time to prepare for gainful employment is *right now!* This is why portfolio development and self-assessment are common themes throughout this worktext. You will analyze and build upon strengths. You will also identify areas that need improvement with a corresponding action plan.

This will not be a passive journey, and you will be expected to be an active participant in this process. This worktext has integrated exercises designed to complement and reinforce the topic under discussion. You will be instructed to *stop* and complete those exercises to further develop the concept. This integrated worktext will then assist you in developing a "portfolio" that will showcase who you are and what you can do.

DEVELOPING PORTFOLIOS

The difference between ordinary and extraordinary is that little extra.

- Author Unknown

During a focus group discussion conducted by the National Center on Education, business personnel were asked about assessment and hiring practices. Many agreed with one person who stated, "When I'm considering an applicant for a job, I want them to be able to show me some examples of schoolwork and what they can do . . . the trouble is, I don't see many students who can present themselves like that."

Of course, this quote will *not* pertain to you. You will be able to showcase your talents and land that job or that seat in the school of your choice. Developing an active portfolio within this worktext will ensure your success. Although portfolios may be somewhat new to classrooms, for years artists, actors, models, journalists, writers, and academicians have been successfully using this concept.

What is a portfolio, and what can it do for you? First, there are many answers to what a portfolio is and what kinds of things should go into its development. One definition states that a portfolio is a systematic and continuous process that continually changes as the learner grows and develops his or her literary and personal skills. This definition seems very technical and not very personal.

Simply stated, a portfolio is a collection of the learner's *work* that can demonstrate his or her progress. For example, an artist's portfolio may contain representative samples of the artist's art. These art samples will be selected to show the artist's talents, styles, and growth. As you work through this worktext, you will learn things that will help you develop skills and gain knowledge that can be presented in your portfolio. The portfolio will become a powerful and friendly tool to help you develop.

Questions abound as to who should have input into the portfolio, how it should be set up, who should review it, how it is to be evaluated, and so on. The author has chosen to make a *user-friendly* portfolio that is highly integrated within a worktext. If the portfolio is to work, it must engage and motivate you in relevant learning activities.

The main goal is to promote active learners who can assess and examine their growth over time. Additional goals that the portfolio will accomplish include:

- Helping students and teachers develop and evaluate meaningful goals
- Assisting students in self-assessment skills
- Creating action plans for development and improvement
- Developing a sense of process and organizational skills
- Enhancing written and oral communication skills
- Emphasizing student responsibility in teaching and learning
- Linking curriculum instruction and assessment to the school and community

Teachers, parents, peers, or school administrators can have input into your portfolio. However, you should organize it and make sure it is showing how you are developing and improving. For example, your worktext will help you develop long-range career and educational goals. These would be good to include in your portfolio. These goals may change over time and need updating, but they will give you a focus or direction as to where you are going. The worktext will also help you to develop a powerful résumé that will serve as a keystone of your portfolio.

SECTION 1

Communicating with Yourself: Achieving Personal Excellence

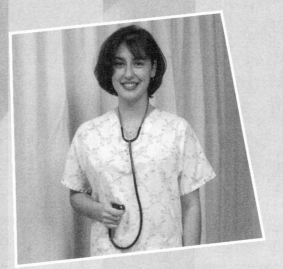

This section focuses on *you!* Only you can ensure that you achieve personal and professional excellence. Therefore, the most important personal relationship you must establish is with yourself.

We all know how crucial good communication skills can be in our relationships with others. But what about communication within ourselves? Positive self-communication is the "foundation" upon which to build a successful personal and professional life.

Therefore, the focus of this section will be on self-examination and self-assessment. You will get to know who you are and how you think. You will then develop action plans to fully realize your personal and professional excellence.

CHAPTER 1

Study Skills: Laying the Foundation

OBJECTIVES

Upon completion of this chapter, you should be able to:

- Relate the importance of good study skill habits to your personal success.
- Perform an assessment of your current study skills and formulate a plan for improvement.

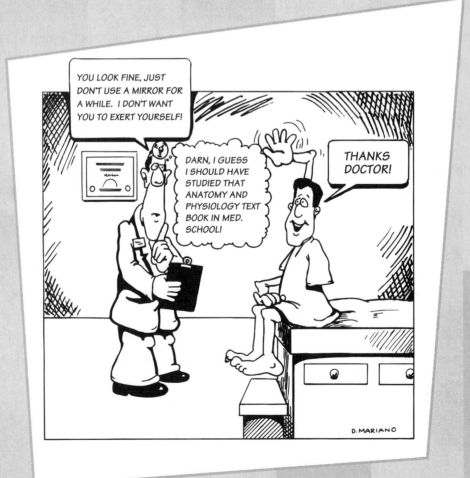

KEY TERMS

acronyms
classical conditioning

critical thinking
mnemonics

INTRODUCTION

Study skills are crucial, so the study skills section is presented first. Even though this is a small chapter, it is critical for your success. Therefore, spend the initial time and effort to lay a solid foundation upon which to build your success.

An initial investment of time and effort in improving study skills will pay off in a big way. It will help you not only with this course, but also with all the current and future courses you take. This chapter discusses five important ingredients that help make studying successful. Activities are given at the end of this chapter to reinforce these concepts.

One of the key things for my success was education.
- Former Boston Celtics Star Bill Russell
(The Michael Jordan of the author's generation)

DAILY PREPARATION

There is *no* substitute for daily preparation. On the surface, it may seem as if this will take a lot of time, but if done correctly, it will actually save a tremendous amount of time. Daily preparation includes developing a schedule plan that budgets your time. This allows you to use the whole day, to do things in proper order, to reduce the confusion in your life, and to have a better sense of accomplishment.

Do not be discouraged if your first few schedules do not work well. Build in some flexibility. Do not forget to schedule relaxation and recreational time; these are important also. Studies show you learn more in three 30-minute sessions than in one 2-hour session. Therefore, studying notes over shorter periods in more frequent intervals is more effective than long cramming sessions. Use 1 hour as your *maximum* study time without a break.

PICK A GOOD TIME AND PLACE OF STUDY

The time you choose to study is very important. It may not be the same time for all of us. Some people are "morning people"; whereas others are not. We all have different biological clocks, so try to schedule times when you are most alert and focused.

The place you choose to study is also important. Ideally, it should be the same place each time so that you "connect" this place to studying and consequently become focused. It should have minimal or no distractions and good lighting. The table or desk should have only the tools of study and not pictures or mementos that may lead to daydreaming.

Have you ever heard of **classical conditioning**? The term came from an experiment performed on dogs. In this experiment, a bell was rung and dogs were then fed meat. The meat caused the dogs to salivate. Again and again, experimenters would ring a bell and feed the dogs. After much repetition, the dogs connected the ringing of the bell to the meat. A bell only had to be rung for the dogs to salivate, even if they were not given meat. What is the purpose of telling you this story other than making you hungry or grossing you out?

When you study in bed and then go to sleep repeatedly, you soon connect studying to sleeping. Every time you begin to study (even in midafternoon), you may begin to yawn and not be as focused. You are conditioning yourself to connect studying to sleeping. Simply avoid studying before sleeping because you will not be as focused and therefore will be less effective. Besides, studying in bed may interfere with your ability to get a good night's sleep.

Classical conditioning can also be used to your advantage in health care. Repeated positive interactions and therapies with a patient will "classically condition" the patient to feel good each time he or she sees you.

USE GOOD STUDY HABITS

Take good, accurate, legible notes. Remember that the purpose of taking notes is to get key points from textbooks and lectures, not to write every word that is said or written. Listen much and write a little.

It is important to be prepared to take notes when class begins by having your notebook, pen, and any handouts or readings at hand. Try to participate actively and constructively in class discussions and do not hesitate to ask questions. Pay attention not only to what the teacher is saying but also to how he or she is saying it. For example, if the teacher says "to summarize" or "the main points are," then this material should be written down along with anything that is written on the board or screen.

Instead of highlighting the chapter, outline your chapters so that you can make the connection from your brain to the pencil. This is

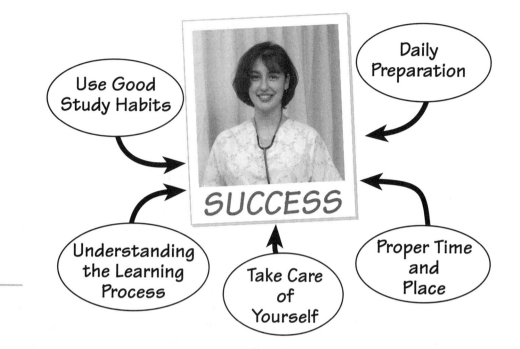

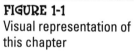

FIGURE 1-1
Visual representation of this chapter

what you will need to do when taking the test. Outlining may initially take longer than highlighting, but you will learn the material better. Outlining actually saves studying time in the long run. Review your lecture and outline notes frequently.

Also make diagrams and pictures to help visualize concepts within your outline. The more you can "see it," the better you can understand relationships or how it all fits together. See Figure 1–1 for a visual representation of this chapter.

Also, periodically ask yourself questions about what you have just read. If you cannot answer these questions, you probably are losing interest and need to take a short break and become more focused.

Study with a friend and explain concepts to each other. Each time you explain something, the oral recitation reinforces your understanding. You will soon learn that there is no better way to learn something than to teach it aloud to someone else.

Be responsible and go to class. Read the assigned readings before class. This will also help you begin to develop professional responsibility skills that are critical in health care.

UNDERSTAND THE LEARNING AND TESTING PROCESS

To succeed, it is important to truly "learn" the material and use **critical thinking** skills to assist in problem solving. *Critical thinking* has many definitions, but most emphasize the ability to gather and analyze information in order to solve problems or create new opportunities. Critical thinking is goal oriented and focuses on a purpose.

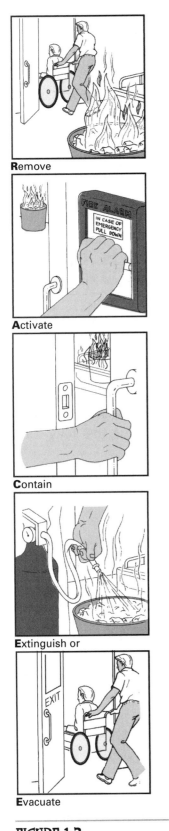

Remove

Activate

Contain

Extinguish or

Evacuate

FIGURE 1-2
An acronym and visual representation to aid in learning the steps to take during a hospital fire

One who can think critically knows how to obtain information, understand it, and apply it. This is a step above merely memorizing information for short-term storage.

Say, for example, you memorize the steps to cardiopulmonary resuscitation (CPR). However, you do not truly understand *why* you need to establish an open airway, or even *how* to actually do it. You may be able to repeat the steps on a pen and paper test and receive a good grade. However, what if in 6 months you are in a situation in which you need to perform CPR on an individual in need? You cannot say, "I had that 6 months ago and I really didn't learn the material."

Education is to encourage thinking skills rather than memorization, but you have to recognize that memory is vital. Memory is used as an index of success because most techniques used to measure learning rely on it. Therefore, a good memory is definitely an asset that you should develop.

Try to memorize only when you are well rested. Also use memorization techniques such as the use of **mnemonics**. Mnemonics are words, rhymes, or formulas that aid your memory. **Acronyms** are one type of mnemonic. An acronym is a word made from the first letters of other words. For example, *HOMES* can help you list the five great lakes (Huron, Ontario, Michigan, Erie, and Superior). The ABCs of CPR remind you that *A* = establish **A**irway, *B* = rescue **B**reathing, and *C* = establish **C**irculation. This helps you better remember the steps and their proper order in a critical situation. Figure 1–2 illustrates an acronym and a picture to aid in learning the steps to take during a hospital fire.

You can also use rhymes or formulas to assist memory. For example, "Spring forward, fall back" helps us remember to adjust our clocks accordingly for daylight savings time. You can also make up silly stories to help remember facts. In fact, often the sillier the story, the easier it is to remember.

When taking examinations, the best advice is to be prepared. If you have prepared daily, you should have no problem. Studying for the test should be reviewing what you already know.

Know what type of test you are taking. With an objective examination (multiple choice, true/false), be sure you understand all directions first. With objective examinations, usually your first idea about the answer is your best. If it is an essay examination (short answer), survey the questions, plan your time, and give time to questions in proportion to their value.

Some people develop their own test-taking strategies. They may do all the easy questions first and then return to the more difficult ones. Make sure you mark the questions you skipped or you may forget to return to them. Finally, do not destroy your old examinations—keep them and learn from them!

TAKE CARE OF YOURSELF

Learning requires a healthy mind, body, and attitude. It is important to exercise your brain to stay mentally fit, but it is also important to stay physically fit. Eating right, exercising several times a week, and staying free of drugs will make you feel better and enhance your ability to learn. There may be times you must study when sick, tired, or fatigued. Begin these study sessions with slow rhythmic breathing. This helps you relax and in turn improves concentration. Remember to get sufficient rest, especially before examinations.

SUMMARY

Study skills are a critical element of your current and future success. The five key ingredients to effective study skills are preparing daily, choosing the proper time and place, using good study habits, understanding the learning process, and taking care of yourself. Taking care of your physical self is crucial for your optimal mental functioning.

LEARNER:

Go to page 8 and complete the Critical Thinking and Application Activities 1–1 through 1–10.

Why These Activities Are Important to You

The importance of good study skill habits cannot be overemphasized. However, you must realize and believe in their importance in order to invest the initial time to establish these skills. These skills will help you improve in all your classes, which will help you get into a better school or obtain a better job. Of course, this then means you will have a better life for yourself and your loved ones. See how it all starts here!

CRITICAL THINKING AND APPLICATION ACTIVITIES

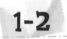 **Why Should You Commit?**

Make a list of five specific things good study skill habits can do for you.

Keep me organized

Help me retain information

Help me learn more efficiently

Making sure I have free time so I don't over do it

Help keeping myself healthy

1-2 **Developing Your Study Schedule**

This chapter discusses five ingredients that will help develop your skills. Let us work on each individually.

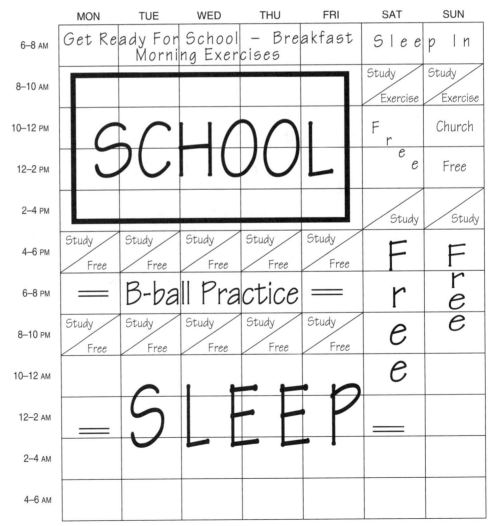

FIGURE 1-3
A sample study schedule

DAILY PREPARATION

Attempt to make a weekly schedule that sets aside time for study. Allow each study block a maximum of 1 hour. Do not forget to add your recreational activities. It may take several schedules before you get all the bugs out. Also, this is just a guide; you must always have flexibility for unexpected events.

The key is to set aside enough study time to properly prepare and stick to a schedule that works for you. Even if you have all your work done, do not skip a study block. Instead, review your notes or quiz yourself.

Figure 1–3 shows a sample schedule. Remember, only you can determine the schedule that is right for your life. Using Figure 1–4, make your own study schedule. Photocopy the blank schedule, so you have several extras. Now attempt to follow this schedule and modify it accordingly until you develop a schedule that works for you. You are encouraged to work with teachers, family members, and friends to help develop and modify the schedule. Post your final schedule in your *special* study place.

	MON	TUE	WED	THU	FRI	SAT	SUN
6–8 AM	Get Ready For the Day		& Care For		Doggies	WORK	WORK
8–10 AM		Phlebotomy	Free time				
10–12 PM	Study		OR study		Computer Essentials		
12–2 PM	Health Care Relations	Study	Health Care Relations Study	Patient Care Techniques Study			
2–4 PM	Patient Care Lab						
4–6 PM	WORK	WORK	WORK	WORK	WORK		
6–8 PM							
8–10 PM	♥	♥	♥	♥	♥		
10–12 AM	Free Time						
12–2 AM	— S L E E P —						
2–4 AM							
4–6 AM							

FIGURE 1-4
Fill in your study schedule

1-3   Finding the Right Time and Place

Assess your current place of study by answering the following questions. Be critical and honestly circle the response that best answers the question.

1. Do you study in the same place each time?   (Sometimes)   Always   Never
2. Is it quiet where you study?   Sometimes   (Always)   Never
3. Are the conditions and lighting comfortable?   Sometimes   (Always)   Never
4. Do you have all the tools (e.g., pencils, rulers,
   computer, paper) you need to study at this place?   Sometimes   (Always)   Never

How well did you do? It does not matter as long as you were honest. Remember this is an assessment of where you are now. Your eventual goal should be to have all your responses be *Always*. If they are now, great! If not, you need to develop an action plan to make all the responses an *Always* in the near future.

1-4   Developing Action Plans

For each question in Activity 1–3 that did not have an *Always* response, develop an action plan that states specifically what you need to do to make the response *Always* in the future. Include a statement about when it will be accomplished. A sample action plan is shown in Figure 1–5. Now complete your action plans.

FIGURE 1-5
A sample action plan

> **Date of plan:** 10-10-05
>
> **Goal:** to improve my study environment
>
> **Plan:** I will improve the lighting in my room by adding a desk lamp. In addition, I will clean my study desk and organize my work area.
>
> **Date accomplished:** 10-20-05
>
> **Evaluation:** This has improved the study area. However, I need to get a higher-watt lightbulb to see better.

Your action plan(s):

Date of plan: Sept.

Goal: Improve my study habits. Commiting to getting it done and not rushing.

Plan: Following a stict schedule and following it.

Date accomplished: _____

Evaluation: _____

Remember to implement and evaluate your plans!

1-5   Developing Good Study Habits

Take a sample chapter from an assigned reading and outline the material. Remember to focus on key points. A sample outline of the study skills section in your textbook is provided.

SAMPLE OUTLINE

STUDY SKILLS

Five Ingredients for Success

A. Prepare daily.

    1. Make up study schedule that works for me.

    2. Keep study sessions to 30–60 minutes.

B. Pick good time and place to study.

    1. *Do not* study in bed.

    2. Choose place with minimal distractions.

    3. Have good lighting.

    4. Make sure table or desk has only needed study tools.

C. Use good study habits.

    1. Take good notes (accurate and legible).

    2. Outline chapters instead of highlighting.

    3. Periodically review notes.

    4. Teach aloud to others.

D. Understand the learning process.

    1. Try to "truly learn the material" and use memorization only as an aid.

    2. Use acronyms (words made from first letter of other words).

    3. Use other memory aids (mnemonics) such as rhymes or stories.

    4. Be prepared for types of examinations and review old tests.

E. Take care of yourself.

    1. Eat right, exercise, and stay drug free.

    2. Get plenty of rest, especially before an examination.

1-6   Helping Memory Skills

UNDERSTAND THE LEARNING AND TESTING PROCESS

This chapter stresses the importance of learning versus memorization. However, it discusses that a good memory is an essential ingredient to the learning process. Let us do some mental gymnastics to build your memory capabilities.

An acronym is a word that comes from the first letters of other words. For example, the treatment for a sprain is to **R**est, **E**levate the sprain, put **I**ce on it, and **C**ompress the effected area. To help you remember this treatment, you can form the following acronym:

    R: Rest

    I : Ice

    C: Compression

    E: Elevate

This could easily help you remember this for a test or when you have to put it into use in a tense situation.

See if you can come up with an acronym for the following:

1. The types of cuts are punctures, incisions, lacerations, and abrasions.

   Acronym: _Pail_

2. A nursing progress note consists of four main parts: A subjective response from the patient, objective patient information, patient assessment, and a plan of action. We discuss what each of these areas means in depth later. For now, see if you can come up with an easy way to remember subjective, objective, assessment, and plan.

   Acronym: _Paint over area_

3. These notes have been expanded to include intervention and evaluation. What could these notes be now called?

   Acronym: _Paint over area inside exit_

Not all acronyms spell a perfect word. For example, the four main types of tissues within the body are epithelial, muscular, nervous, and connective tissue. One acronym is C-MEN. You may also need to add vowels to form recognizable terms.

You can also use mnemonics such as rhymes or formulas to help your memory. For example, "mother very early made johnny sit up near papa" tells you the planets within our solar system in order from the sun. You may not know which *M* is for Mercury and which is for Mars, but use your intuition. Mercury is in a thermometer and relates to heat and therefore is closer (hotter) to the sun. Your memory combined with your thinking skills can be very powerful.

Try to make a mnemonic up for the following:

1. Lines of a treble clef: E, G, B, D, F

   Mnemonic: _Every Good Boy Deserves Fudge_

2. Colors in the spectrum: red, orange, yellow, green, blue, indigo, and violet

   Mnemonic: _Roygbiv_

3. The body's vital signs: pulse, respirations, temperature, and blood pressure

   Mnemonic: _PRTB_

1-7 Do You Take Care of Yourself?

A future chapter discusses the importance of proper exercise, nutrition, and healthy living habits. In that chapter, you will make a thorough assessment and develop an action plan for a healthier you. Circle the answer to the following general questions and make an action plan for each "yes" answer(s).

1. Do you feel tired during the day when you are studying?   Yes   (No)

2. Do you take any mood-altering drugs? Remember alcohol and cigarettes are included in this category.   (Yes)   No

3. Do you forget to exercise during the week?   (Yes)   No

4. Do you eat a diet that is heavy in fats and "junk food"?   Yes   (No)

Your action plan:

Date of plan: _Sept_

Goal: _Cut back or quit smoking_

Eat healthy

Plan: _____
_____
_____

Date accomplished: _____
Evaluation: _____
_____
_____

Your action plan:
Date of plan: _____
Goal: _____
_____
_____

Plan: _____
_____
_____

Date accomplished: _____
Evaluation: _____
_____
_____

Remember to implement and evaluate your plans!

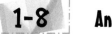 **1-8** ## Ancient Wisdom

Explain how the following proverb relates to studying and learning.

> **T**ell me and I'll forget, show me and I may remember, but involve me and I'll understand.
> — Chinese Proverb

Getting involved with hands on is the best way to remember anything you need to retain in your memory.
_____
_____

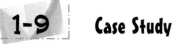 **Case Study**

Karla was an excellent student in high school, who in her own words "hardly ever took a book home or studied." However, she is now in a health care program, which is much faster paced and more demanding than high school. She can't seem to keep up with all the extra readings and is doing poorly on her exams.

What do you think is the main reason for this good student now performing poorly?

Her old (non) study habits are hard to break. She needs to change them and commit.

What would you suggest she do to turn this situation around in a positive direction?

Putting in the effort is worth the reward.

 Internet Activity

Using Internet search engines, try to find additional material on studying that can help you and your fellow students. Some suggested keywords are: study skills, memory aids, and test taking. Write down something new that you found and can share.

Congratulations on your work concerning study skills. The time you invested will pay great dividends in your life. Use these skills in this and other courses, and they will serve you well.

CHAPTER 2

Personal and Professional Characteristics for Success

OBJECTIVES

Upon completion of this chapter, you should be able to:

Define "success" in your own terms.

Relate concepts of self-esteem, values, and attitudes toward *your* life.

Incorporate a positive and professional attitude in dealing with others.

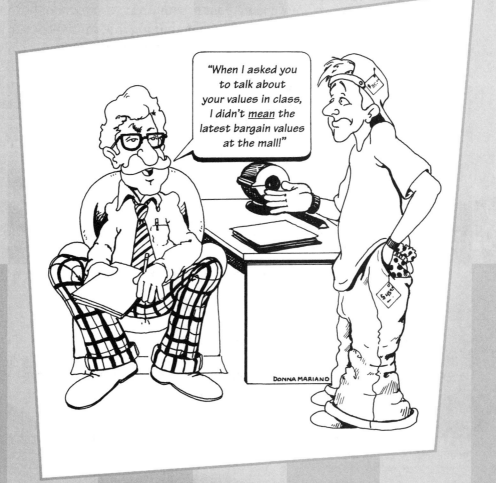

"When I asked you to talk about your values in class, I didn't <u>mean</u> the latest bargain values at the mall!"

DONNA MARIANO

KEY TERMS

caring attitude

competency

endorphins

negative attitude

positive attitude

profession

self-confident attitude

self-esteem

self-motivation

service industry

tact

trustworthy attitude

values

victim attitude

INTRODUCTION

You can get lost in all the *self* terms. For example, people talk about self-esteem, self-concept, self-responsibility, self-management, self-awareness, self-help, and so on. It is easy to get lost in all the terms. Where do you start so that you are not overwhelmed?

I think the answer is **self-motivation**. Self-motivation is one of the characteristics that most influences a person's behavior. In other words, do you want something badly enough to put in the work to achieve your goals? That is something that cannot be taught but must come from within. However, having that motivation or internal drive is not enough. You must combine motivation with an awareness of yourself and develop certain skills to realize your full potential. If you have the internal drive, this chapter gives you the awareness. The remaining chapters in this section build on this awareness and give you life skills to achieve your goals.

Although I stated you cannot teach self-motivation, you can foster an environment where it will develop. The first step is to look at how you feel about yourself and work on your internal environment.

What Do YOU Think?

What Is Success?

The following is attributed to the American writer Ralph Waldo Emerson.

Success

To laugh often and much; to win the respect of intelligent people and the affection of children; to earn the appreciation of honest critics and endure the betrayal of false friends; to appreciate beauty; to find the best in others; to leave the world a bit better, whether by a healthy child, a garden patch or a redeemed social condition; to know even one life has breathed easier because you have lived.

This is to have succeeded.

What do you think about Mr. Emerson's definition? Write a paragraph about what has the most meaning to you in his writing.

LEARNER:

Go to page 32 and complete the Critical Thinking and Application Activities 2–1 and 2–2.

SELF-ESTEEM

What is **self-esteem**? Simply stated, it is how *you* feel about yourself. Other words for self-esteem are self-belief or self-concept. Regardless of the term used, this is probably one of the most important questions you need to answer in your life. The way you feel about yourself affects every aspect of your life. In fact, many studies show that there is a direct relationship between self-esteem and academic performance. Simply put, the better you feel about yourself, the better you will do in school. The better you do in school, the better your chance for a successful and fulfilling life. In addition, having good self-esteem enhances your ability to interact with others in a positive way. This is a prime ingredient for any health care provider. Which photo in Figure 2–1 demonstrates positive self-esteem? Which of these health care workers would you want to care for you?

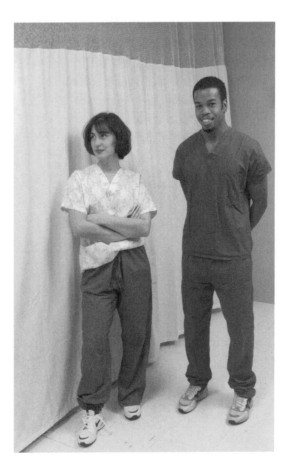

FIGURE 2-1
Who looks more professional?

Self-esteem is shaped by your **values**. Values are what you believe in. They are your own thoughts and feelings about yourself. They are comprised of the following:

1. What you think
2. How you feel
3. How you act based on how you think and feel

For example, you may *value* competency in an individual. **Competency** means someone is capable of doing something well. Therefore, you "think" as a future health care professional that you should be competent. Emotionally, you "feel" good when you are competent at a procedure and uncomfortable when you are not. Finally, you "act" on these feelings. You may practice a procedure more and more until you become comfortable with it.

How did your values come about? They formed as you developed. Your values were (and are still being) influenced by family, friends, teachers, and the society in which you live.

Attitudes arise from values. For example, you value the concept of honesty. Therefore, you should be honest in your words and deeds. Because you value honesty, you will not lie in your relationships with others. You will be viewed as someone who can be trusted and be truthful in any situation. Figure 2–2 shows how positive values can be shaped.

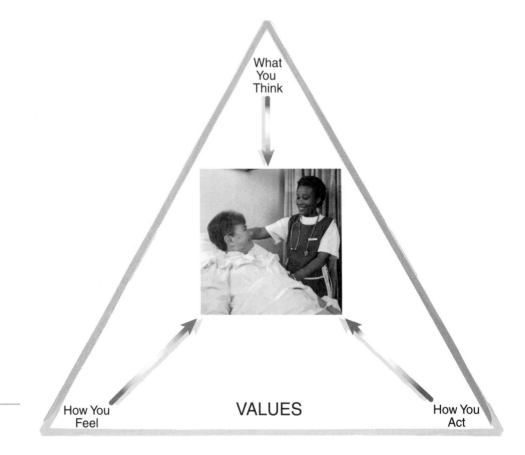

FIGURE 2-2
How values arise

SELF-CONFIDENT ATTITUDE

A **self-confident attitude** is important for health care professionals (and actually everyone). Being self-confident means you know yourself inside and out. You have assessed your strengths and weaknesses and are confident in what you can do. You believe in your ability to do things and make things happen in a positive manner.

Another component of a self-confident attitude is the ability to be assertive. An appropriately assertive and self-confident attitude is important in health care. For example, what if a physician prescribes a medication dosage that you are sure is incorrect? Do you give the dosage because the doctor prescribed it? Or do you call and double-check, even though you may get yelled at for questioning the physician's orders? What would you do in this situation?

Here is one final word to the wise. Anything can be taken to an extreme. Assertiveness taken to the extreme becomes aggressiveness. Self-confidence taken to the extreme becomes obnoxiousness.

TEST Yourself

How Assertive Are You?

1. I can express my feelings easily.	Always	Sometimes	Never
2. I tell a person when I do not like what he or she said or did.	Always	Sometimes	Never
3. I tell people what to do directly.	Always	Sometimes	Never
4. I am not embarrassed to tell someone what I think of them.	Always	Sometimes	Never
5. I do not think people take advantage of me.	Always	Sometimes	Never
6. I am not afraid to tell others the truth about how I feel.	Always	Sometimes	Never
7. I see the necessity of expressing my feelings to someone else.	Always	Sometimes	Never
8. I can say "no" to people without feeling bad.	Always	Sometimes	Never

If you are an assertive person you should have mostly *Always* answers with no *Never* answers. If you do have *Never* answers, this is an area that needs improvement. But how do you improve?

Let us say you answered *Never* to number 8. You fear telling someone no because you think he or she might not like you. How can you overcome this? One way is through role-playing. You can practice with a friend. Remember, to get good at something takes practice. Have your friend assume the role of someone who is asking a favor of you. Imagine that your friend is asking you to work Friday night. However, you have an important date and say no. As in real life, have your friend really not hear you say no and continue to try to persuade you and make you feel guilty, to get a yes response. Practice saying no and not feeling bad with your friend. By practicing in this made-up scenario, you will be better prepared next time it happens to you in real life.

What Do YOU Think?

Do You Walk the Walk or Talk the Talk?

Have you ever heard someone say another person has an "attitude"? This can be good or bad depending on how the person says it or what that person's attitude is when he or she says it. An *attitude* is a state of mind. It is how you feel about a person, object, or situation. Your attitudes can be picked up by others. An attitude can be shown by your outward physical appearance or expressions (body language). Attitudes can come through when you talk and interact with others.

Have you ever heard someone say that another person "walks the walk"? This means the person truly lives his or her values. In this case, personal attitude is consistent with personal values. The person acts the way he or she believes.

But what if someone just "talks the talk"? This means what the person states is his or her values is not consistent with his or her words or deeds. For example, as a health professional, you will be asked to educate your patients on health awareness. Let's say that it is your job to stress the importance of taking care of yourself and taking your medications on time and in a responsible manner. However, you come into the room 10 minutes late smelling of cigarette smoke. Would what you say really be effective? How would you feel if this happened to you?

LEARNER:

Go to page 34 and complete the Critical Thinking and Application Activities 2–3, 2–4, and 2–5.

WHAT IS A PROFESSIONAL ATTITUDE?

You have chosen the health occupations. This is a **service industry**, which means you are providing a service to others. In this case, the others are in great need because their health is vitally important. This is also a **profession**, which means it sets high standards for those who claim to be professional. Therefore, it is important for you to develop the personal and professional attitudes that will make you stand out as a competent health care professional.

Remember a time when you or someone you know interacted with a health care professional? Was he or she professional? What is a professional attitude? The listing of the traits or characteristics of a health care professional can be extensive. However, they can be grouped into three categories as to what most people expect from a professional health care provider. People expect to be treated by a *trustworthy, caring,* and *competent* individual. These characteristics and attitudes should become part of your personality.

TRUSTWORTHY ATTITUDE

Patients, coworkers, and supervisors must trust you. Patients are literally placing their most precious possession, their lives, in your

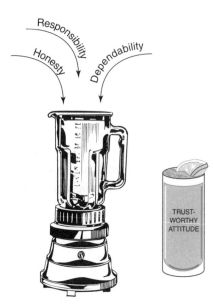

FIGURE 2-3
The vital ingredients of a trustworthy attitude

hands. Many things that are said during their stay could be highly confidential. They must be able to depend on you in their time of need.

A **trustworthy attitude**, Figure 2–3, consists of three main ingredients:

- Honesty
- Dependability
- Responsibility

Honesty means to be truthful. This will help establish trust in a patient relationship. Dependability means people can count on you to be there. They can depend on your arriving on time for their treatment. This includes being on time for school and work. Your attendance record is an important reflection on your motivation. Responsibility is fulfilling your obligation to do something. It also means you are accountable and take responsibility for what you have done and how well you have done it.

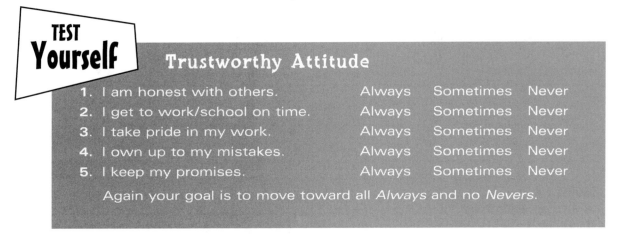

TEST Yourself

Trustworthy Attitude

1. I am honest with others.	Always	Sometimes	Never
2. I get to work/school on time.	Always	Sometimes	Never
3. I take pride in my work.	Always	Sometimes	Never
4. I own up to my mistakes.	Always	Sometimes	Never
5. I keep my promises.	Always	Sometimes	Never

Again your goal is to move toward all *Always* and no *Nevers*.

CARING ATTITUDE

Have you heard of TLC? It stands for tender loving care. To some, it may sound wimpy, but consider this. You are in a strange environment (hospital), and you have just been told you have a critical medical problem that requires immediate treatment. The chances are 50/50 you will survive. You are frightened and you have several questions. No matter who you are, a caring and concerned health care professional would certainly be welcomed at this time.

A **caring attitude**, Figure 2–4, comprises the following:

- Sincerity and empathy
- Respect
- Tact

Sincerity means you *genuinely* care about another individual. Patients are highly perceptive and can spot a phony quickly. They are usually so focused on their caregiver that they can pick up on someone "acting" like they care. A measure of one's sincerity is his or her ability to empathize with patients. Empathy is the ability to identify with and understand another person's feelings, situation, and motives. It means you can understand and are compassionate toward what another person is going through. It also means not being judgmental.

Respect means you treat others with consideration. It means you are kind and courteous about the patient's needs. You do not burst in while a patient is taking a bath or having an uncomfortable procedure done. You respect the patient's privacy and territory. Always remember it is the patient's room, and you are the guest. Say please and thank you. Treat people with patience and tolerance. Calmly react to any given patient or situation.

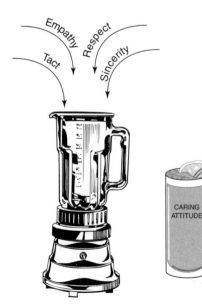

FIGURE 2-4
The vital ingredients of a caring attitude

Tact is rubbing out another's mistake instead of rubbing it in.

- Author Unknown

Tact is a term often used in dealing with patients. Tact means being considerate of the feelings of others in difficult situations. It is saying or doing the right thing. This is a difficult skill in the hospital environment and requires a lot of practice.

Many people start off on the wrong foot by using a "you" statement to tell a person what he or she should think, feel, or do. Would you be offended if someone told you how to feel, what to think, or what to do? One way to be more tactful is to use an "I" statement to tell someone what you feel or need. For example, instead of telling a patient "*you* don't know how to take your medication correctly," say "*I* think you would greatly benefit from taking your medication like this." The second statement does not put down or blame the patient.

TEST Yourself — Caring Attitude

	Always	Sometimes	Never
1. I get along with others.	Always	Sometimes	Never
2. I treat everyone equally.	Always	Sometimes	Never
3. I am polite and courteous.	Always	Sometimes	Never
4. I can make people feel comfortable in uncomfortable situations.	Always	Sometimes	Never
5. I can "feel" for someone else or their situation.	Always	Sometimes	Never
6. I respect other's privacy.	Always	Sometimes	Never

Again, *Always* responses should be your goal.

COMPETENT ATTITUDE

You certainly want someone who is treating you for an illness or accident to know what he or she is doing. You must have a competent attitude so that your patients will have faith in your abilities to bring them through a crisis.

Competency means that you have the ability to perform a certain task. You are proficient. Proficiency means you can accurately, and in a timely manner, follow the approved steps and procedures to get the job done well. A competent attitude, Figure 2–5, consists of the following ingredients:

- Willingness to learn
- Willingness to change
- Acceptance of criticism
- Enthusiasm for learning

To be competent in the health care profession, you must be self-motivated and have a desire and willingness to learn.

You must be willing to learn on a continual basis. New techniques and equipment are constantly being developed. You need to keep up to date and be willing to continue your education to maintain your competency.

Closely related to this is a willingness to change. Health care changes because of research, new inventions, and many other factors. People tend to resist change. However, new research in health care may state a drug is not as effective as once thought because of a mutated virus. We must be willing to change our treatment accordingly for the good of our patients.

A competent person also listens to others' evaluations of his or her interaction with patients or their performance of techniques. We must therefore accept constructive criticism. We learn from our mistakes and the mistakes of others if we have the proper attitude. Constructive (proper) criticism from coworkers, teachers, friends, or patients can help us become better at what we do. After all, this is what we are striving for.

Remember that mistakes are not failures. We all make mistakes and can use them to improve our future performance. When you make a mistake as a health care professional, a specific procedure is

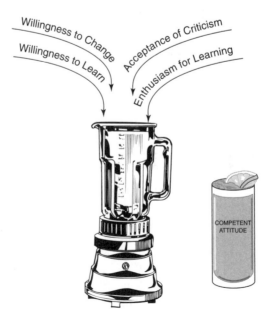

FIGURE 2-5
The vital ingredients of a
competent attitude

followed. Let us say you made a drug medication error. An incident report would be filled out by you and your supervisor. The goal is not to punish but to evaluate why it happened and to prevent future errors. This can lead to overall improvements for workers and patients alike.

Everyone gets criticism. Unfortunately, it is not always done properly or constructively. We will discuss how to give constructive criticism to others in upcoming chapters. For now, however, there are certain behaviors that are unprofessional when being criticized. The following is a list of negative reactions to criticisms. You should *not* do the following:

Get angry

Make excuses

Complain

Blame others

Whine or cry

Criticize your supervisor in turn

Run or walk away

> **W**e must accept finite disappointment, but we must never lose infinite hope.
> — Martin Luther King, Jr.

Finally, enthusiasm for learning and performing the task at hand is important. This does not mean you are enthusiastic because someone is dying and you have to perform cardiopulmonary resuscitation (CPR). Rather, you accept the reality of the situation, and because you have trained well, you are enthusiastic to save a life. Enthusiasm shows as an eagerness or excitement for what you are doing. It helps make the learning go easier. It also helps present a positive attitude. Enthusiasm is a highly contagious condition that is worth getting.

TEST Yourself

Competent Attitude

1. I continually strive to improve.	Always	Sometimes	Never
2. I accept criticism easily.	Always	Sometimes	Never
3. I enjoy learning new skills.	Always	Sometimes	Never
4. I work with enthusiasm.	Always	Sometimes	Never
5. I can accept change.	Always	Sometimes	Never

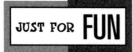

Different societies have different combination of words or expressions that are particular to them. These are called idioms.

Match the idiom with the corresponding attitude it relates to.

1. _____ Perseverance   a. give and take

2. _____ Honesty/directness   b. work like a dog

3. _____ Anger   c. hang in there

4. _____ Hard work   d. on top of the world

5. _____ Kindness and helpfulness   e. cut the apron strings

6. _____ Cooperation   f. lay your cards on the table

7. _____ Compromise   g. two heads are better than one

8. _____ Independence   h. give you the shirt off my back

9. _____ Happiness   i. breathing space

10. _____ Privacy   j. hot-headed

LEARNER:

Go to page 36 and complete the Critical Thinking and Application Activities 2–6 and 2–7.

POSITIVE AND NEGATIVE ATTITUDES

Whether you think you can or think you can't— you're probably right.

- Henry Ford

Your attitude influences how you think and feel about life. This in turn determines your behaviors and how well you interact or get along with others. You have two choices. Do you want to have a positive or negative attitude?

In less than 30 seconds, you have made an impression on others. A first impression is the opinion that others make about you as a result of the image you present. If your first impression is positive, they will probably want to get to know you. So what will you present?

Is the glass half-empty or half-full? Is the weather partly sunny or partly cloudy? Is this going to be a good day or a bad day? What would you pick? Your answer depends on your attitude. A person with a positive attitude would say the glass is half-full, it is a partly sunny day, and the day is going to be good. Realistically, things may happen that may not make it a perfect day, but a positive person will make the best of it, maintaining a **positive attitude** and being upbeat, optimistic, and cheerful, even in the face of adversity. The positive person will enjoy the day and be excited about what he or she is doing. Others will enjoy being around that person. With a positive attitude, you will convey the three professional attitudes discussed previously. This will put others at ease and help them in their recovery process. In addition, your coworkers will enjoy working with you.

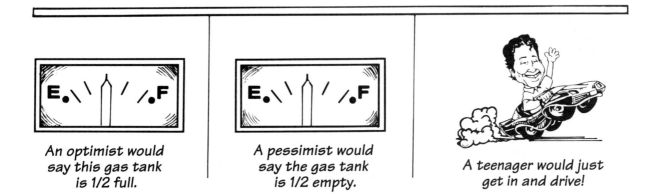

An optimist would say this gas tank is 1/2 full.

A pessimist would say the gas tank is 1/2 empty.

A teenager would just get in and drive!

However, a person with a **negative attitude** will see a half-empty glass and be angry about the partly cloudy day. This attitude conveys unhappiness and is not very pleasant to be around. Pessimists will be sure it is going to be a bad day and will complain often and blame others for their misery. Is this the type of person you would want to spend time with?

CHARACTERISTICS OF POSITIVE ATTITUDES

Thinking positively can enhance every aspect of your life. It could be one of the most important attitudes that will relate to your success. However, learning to think positively is like learning to do anything else—it takes knowledge and practice.

So what are some of the characteristics of a person with a positive attitude? We already discussed many of them. A willingness to learn and accept changes, enthusiasm, and respect for others. A positive outlook on life shows through in your body language. A friendly facial expression reflects a positive attitude. It also shows that you are calm and in control of the situation.

Positive people are also open to others' viewpoints and backgrounds. This means being able to at least consider new ideas, opinions, and different cultural backgrounds. You may not agree, but you listen and do not judge the individual. Most people would agree that this is how they would want to be treated. This willingness to be open is also a sign of your maturity and flexibility.

Positive people accept responsibility and constructive criticism. They admit their mistakes without blaming others or making excuses. Positive people can do the things necessary to correct their errors and learn how to avoid repeating them.

Positive people also have a good sense of humor. Humor is important in health care for many reasons. It helps the healing process for many patients. It also helps relieve the stress of many tense situations that can occur in the hospital environment. However, humor must be used at the appropriate time and place or it could also be offensive.

What Do YOU Think?

Humor in Medicine

LAUGHTER is contagious . . . start an epidemic.
- Author Unknown

It may seem strange to talk about humor in the medical professions. However, much scientific research is now being done to determine the benefits of humor in the healing process. Some research suggests that laughter helps the immune system become better in warding off illness. This is not to say that humor therapy and positive emotions can replace medical treatment. They simply can enhance the medical treatment and the body's positive response. Let's look at the process of laughter.

A good laugh has been shown to increase the heart rate and improve blood circulation. Epinephrine levels in the blood also rise. This is the body's arousal hormone and stimulates the release of **endorphins**. Endorphins are the body's natural painkillers. In addition, other immunologic responses are increased. Finally, the entire respiratory system gets a workout along with our facial muscles. These are some physiologic outcomes of laughter, but what about the psychological effects?

Humor has been shown to relieve tension and lessen anxiety. This is important in the sometimes frightening hospital environment. Humor can also help one's self-image and stimulate creativity when appropriately used. Some smoking cessation programs are now using humor therapy to help substitute humor as a coping strategy for the addictive and dangerous nicotine. In Chapter 1, you were encouraged to use humor in making up silly stories to aid your learning. So use humor when you can, and remember that what is learned with humor is not readily forgotten. To help you, we have included some fictitious mixed-up medical terminology.

Barium: what you do when CPR fails

Cesarean section: a district in Rome

Coma: a punctuation mark

Dilate: to live long

Fester: quicker

GI series: baseball games between teams of soldiers

Hangnail: a coat hook

Medical staff: a doctor's cane

Morbid: a higher offer

Outpatient: a person who has fainted

Protein: in favor of young people

Serology: study of English knighthood

Tablet: a small table

Tumor: an extra pair

Urine: opposite of you're out

Varicose veins: veins that are very close together

NEGATIVE ATTITUDES

Studies have shown that the average child receives 432 negative messages per day, compared with 32 positive. Many contend these messages are absorbed into our subconscious, internalized, and carried with us. Not a very positive thought.

In addition, negative attitudes can be quite contagious and cause others to join in. Have you ever heard the expression, "One bad apple spoils the whole barrel"? A person with a negative attitude is one who does not welcome change or accept imperfections in others. Such a person often blames others for his or her "bad" situation. This type of person is not very pleasant to work with because he or she always has a complaint about someone or something. Having a complaint about a situation is okay. However, a negative person will not offer any positive solutions, yet may continue to stir up the problem. A positive person will properly state the problem and think of ways to make it better.

VICTIM ATTITUDE

The fault, dear Brutus, is not in our stars, but in ourselves.

- Shakespeare, Julius Caesar

The book *The Oz Principle,* by Conners, Smith, and Hickman, states America is in crisis because of a **victim attitude**. It goes on to state that this attitude, which perpetuates helplessness, keeps the person in that victim mode. Granted many people have bad situations, but there is hope for change. You do not need to call a psychic hot line for the answer. The solution lies within yourself.

The Oz Principle states four steps to get out of the victim mode. They are:

See it: Identify the problem.

Own it: Take personal responsibility for it.

Solve it: Identify possible options.

Do it: Pick an option and take action to implement it.

One suggestion would be to add "check it: assess the outcome" to this list as the final step. In other words, evaluate your solution to see how effective it is and modify it accordingly. The Reverend Jesse Jackson, a civil rights leader who grew up in poverty, achieved many great accomplishments because of his belief in the power of a person's attitude. He stated: "I am somebody! If my mind can conceive it, and my heart can believe it, I know I can achieve it!"

CHANGING NEGATIVE ATTITUDES INTO POSITIVE ATTITUDES

There are other ways to change negative attitudes into positive. Have you ever heard of a self-fulfilling prophecy? It means if you believe something strongly enough, it can come true.

For example, if you tell yourself that you will never get organized, you will not. However, you can use this same principle to your advantage by using positive self-talk. Talking to yourself does not mean you are crazy. In fact, talking is slower than thinking and therefore slows your racing mind down. This allows you to be more focused.

Self-talk can boost self-esteem if it is optimistic and positive. Replace negative internal messages such as "I'm not smart enough," with "if I study hard I *can* do well. . . ." Do not dwell on past negative or unpleasant experiences and do not carry grudges. This only depletes your energy and destroys motivation.

Be open and direct with your communications. And remember to lighten up and take care of yourself.

Finally, remember that no one is perfect. For example, many people view anger as a negative emotion. However, a little anger is good. It spurs us on to do better or to right an injustice. Another example is that we all feel sad when tragedy strikes. This is what makes us human. However, taken to extremes, anger can be dangerous and sadness can lead to severe depression.

An important idea to think about is that people do not get you upset, you do! You are the only person who can make you angry or upset or feel bad. *You* feel the way *you* think.

YOU CAN MAKE A DIFFERENCE

The following story is an example of someone making a difference.

The Starfish

There was a young man walking down a deserted beach just before dawn. In the distance he saw a frail old man. As he approached the old man, he saw him picking up stranded starfish and throwing them back into the sea. The young man gazed in wonder as the old man again and again threw the small starfish from the sand to the water. He asked him, "Why do you spend so much energy doing what seems to be a waste of time?" The old man explained that the stranded starfish would die if left in the morning sun. "But there must be thousands of beaches and millions of starfish," exclaimed the young man. "How can your effort make any difference?" The old man looked down at the small starfish in his hand and as he threw it to safety in the sea said . . . "It makes a difference to this one."

What does this story mean to you? Remember you have one precious chance called a lifetime. It is up to you to make the most of every day. Celebrate and be enthusiastic about life. If you make a positive difference in just one person's life, you have done well. Think of how many lives you can touch as a health care professional!

SUMMARY

To be successful, you must begin with good self-esteem and a set of positive values and attitudes. There are certain attitudes that are required of a health care professional.

- A trustworthy attitude develops from being honest, dependable, and responsible.

- A caring attitude is fostered by showing sincerity, empathy, respect, and tact when dealing with patients and coworkers.

- A competent attitude will be demonstrated by your enthusiasm and willingness to learn and accept change, coupled with acceptance of proper criticism.

Finally, a personal positive attitude will greatly influence your future success as a health care professional.

LEARNER:

Go to page 37 and complete the Critical Thinking and Application Activities 2–8, 2–9, 2–10, 2–11, 2–12, and 2–13.

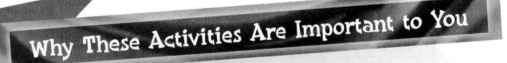

Why These Activities Are Important to You

This chapter is crucial to your success as a health care practitioner. It is also critical for your success in life. It will help you explore your "inner space." We all can improve, but first we need to take a hard look at (assess) who we are in order to see how we can better ourselves.

CRITICAL THINKING AND APPLICATION ACTIVITIES

2-1 Attributes of Success

1. List three people you know personally, whom you consider to be successful.

   a. _____

   b. _____

   c. _____

2. What is it about these individuals that led you to call them successful? Write a short paragraph for each individual to answer this question.

   _____

   _____

   _____

   _____

   _____

   _____

   _____

   _____

   _____

   _____

   _____

   _____

   _____

   _____

   _____

   _____

3. Interview at least one of these individuals and list five reasons why that person thinks he or she is a success.

   a. _____

   b. _____

   c. _____

   d. _____

   e. _____

4. Who are your heroes? Why are they your heroes? Pick one and write all the reasons why you admire this person.

   _____

   _____

Your Own Definition of Success

Everyone has a different definition of what success is. It is important for you to have a clear definition of what you believe is success. It can have many parts to it. Some parts can be short-term and accomplished within a few months or a year, while others may take several years to achieve. For example, hopefully one short-term goal is the successful completion of your health care courses for this year. A long-term goal may be the securing of a professional job in your chosen area. While this is *your* definition, please exercise one caution. Too often in our society, success is equated to money or accumulation of material possessions. Although this may be part of your success goals, try not to make it your sole focus. Look within, for no matter how much your net worth is, it does not mean very much if you are not happy with yourself or your situation.

1. In one paragraph, state your definition of success.

   _____

   _____

   _____

   _____

2. List five characteristics you have that will help you become successful.

   a. _____

   b. _____

   c. _____

   d. _____

   e. _____

3. List two short-term success goals (accomplished within 1 year).

   a. _____

   b. _____

4. List two long-term success goals (accomplished within 5 years).

   a. _____

   b. _____

   NOTE: We will talk more about how to write goals in Chapter 3. For now, just write your goal in your own words.

VALUES

What are your values? How do they shape your attitudes? These are important questions. You may not be happy with all that you find. Congratulations. This means you are working hard and being honest. We all have some values that should be questioned and attitudes that need work. The first step is to assess our values and attitudes and then to improve upon them.

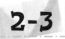

Taking a Look at Yourself

Answer the following general questions.

1. I am good at _____.
2. The three most important things in my life are _____.
3. I want people to remember me as someone who _____.
4. The most important thing someone can do with their life is _____.
5. I like people who _____.
6. I get angry when _____.
7. The most important attitude in a relationship is _____.

The answers to these questions can begin to tell you a little about your attitude.

Your Values

We discussed in this chapter how a value arises from the following:

1. What you think
2. How you feel
3. How you act on those feelings

For each of the values, state how you think, feel, and act in your own words. An example is done for you.

Open-minded: *I "think" open-mindedness is important in dealing with people and situations. I "feel" upset when someone is not open-minded about my opinion. I will "act" to become more open-minded when others disagree or have a different viewpoint.*

Kind: _____

_____

_____

_____

Ambitious: _____

_____

_____

_____

Brave: _____

_____

_____

_____

Cheerful: _____

_____

_____

_____

Competent: _____

_____

_____

_____

Courteous: _____

_____

_____

_____

Forgiving: _____

_____

_____

_____

Helpful: _____

_____

_____

_____

Honest: _____

_____

_____

_____

Open-minded: _____

_____

_____

_____

Responsible: _____

_____

_____

_____

 Your Attitudes

1. List and describe five values or characteristics that you think are important for a self-motivated attitude.

   a. _____

   b. _____

   c. _____

   d. _____

   e. _____

2. You never get a second chance to make a first impression. What attitude would make a good first impression on you?

_____

PROFESSIONAL IMAGE

Although you may not be aware of it, your reputation—the image other people have about you—begins the first moment that you walk into a room. You really never get a second chance to make a first impression. Think of when you or a loved one were treated by medical professionals. What were the characteristics of the people you believed were professional? Were there any contacts that were unprofessional? Let us explore the attitudes that would lead to a professional reputation.

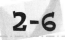 **Professional Attitudes**

1. Describe a situation in which a person's attitude made a difficult situation easier for you.

_____

_____

2. Why is it important to be tactful when dealing with others?

_____

_____

3. How would you gain the trust of a skeptical or withdrawn patient?

_____

_____

 Taking a Look at Yourself

Let us explore some of your characteristics that can enhance a professional image. We talk more about how to take care of yourself in upcoming chapters, but we can begin to get a baseline as to where you are now. Check the items you think you do on a regular basis. Your goal should be to eventually have all the items checked.

1. _____ I take quiet time to clear my mind and recharge my batteries.
2. _____ I take pride in my work.
3. _____ I am on time for school/work.
4. _____ I avoid using slang or jargon terms in conversation.
5. _____ I work on my conversational skills and attempt to enhance my vocabulary.
6. _____ I present proper body language when interacting with others (listen genuinely, make direct eye contact, avoid fidgeting around or tapping my foot or looking at my watch).
7. _____ I do not smoke or chew gum.
8. _____ I dress professionally (clothes are clean, well pressed, and well fitted). The trendy, casual look is good in school, but a more formal professional look is needed on your job and will assist you in commanding the authority you need to deliver health care.
9. _____ I smile and am pleasant to be with.
10. _____ I do not complain all the time.

11. _____ I show a genuine interest in others.

12. _____ I make others feel important by respecting their ideas and giving praise when it is due.

13. _____ I acknowledge other points of view and am willing to change ideas and behaviors when necessary.

14. _____ I am a good listener and I do not gossip.

15. _____ I do not brag or act superior.

16. _____ I accept responsibility for my mistakes and try to correct them.

POSITIVE IMPRESSIONS

In less than 30 seconds, you have made an impression on others. A first impression is the opinion that others make about you as a result of the image that you present at your introduction. If your first impression is positive, they will probably want to get to know you.

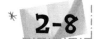

First Impressions

1. How do first impressions affect your patient interaction?

   _____

   _____

2. List five things you can do to make a positive first impression with a patient or a coworker. (For example, a smile and a firm handshake.)

   a. _____

   b. _____

   c. _____

   d. _____

   e. _____

2-9   Positive Attitudes

1. What positive attitudes do you find appealing? Why?

   _____

   _____

   _____

2. What are your favorite songs and TV shows? Do many of them have positive messages?

   _____

   _____

   _____

3. List 10 positive things about yourself. Jot down the first things that come to mind; these are usually your truest feelings. Make sure they are just what you think is wonderful about you, not what others think.

a. _____   f. _____

b. _____   g. _____

c. _____   h. _____

d. _____   i. _____

e. _____   j. _____

4. Make a star by the top three you would want to be remembered by. Now think about qualities you did not list. Now pick two professional qualities you want to work on and describe how you will work on these.

_____

_____

Had I asked you to list your negatives, would this list have been easier to make? If so, you are not alone, but you must work on breaking the negative cycle.

*2-10   Using Positive Self-Talk

Complete the following statements with how you would talk to yourself.

Example

When I realize I have made a mistake, I tell myself that *it is okay, everyone makes a mistake. The important thing is to learn from my mistakes, move on, and improve.*

1. When I am criticized, I_____.
2. When nothing I do seems to be right, I _____.
3. When I do something good, I _____.
4. When I get angry, I _____.
5. When I do something that I think is wrong, I_____.
6. When I have a good idea, I _____.
7. When I feel anxious about something, I_____.

What negative attitudes bother you the most? Why?

_____

_____

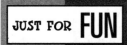 Here are some attitudes that you do not want to be associated with.

The tank: confrontational and aggressive

The sniper: identifies everyone's weakness and talks behind others' backs

The grenade: explodes suddenly about things that have nothing to do with the circumstances

The know-it-all: seldom in doubt, has low tolerance for anyone who disagrees with him or her, and if something goes wrong, it was somebody else's fault

The yes person: quick to agree, slow to deliver—unkept commitments and broken promises but always says yes to please

The maybe person: puts off decisions till it's too late—never commits

The no person: deadly to morale, able to defeat great ideas in a single syllable—discouraging

The whiner: overwhelmed by an unfair world—no one measures up to his or her standard of perfection

The denier: says there is no problem—ignore or deny it and it will go away

GOOD HABITS

Good habits are the ways of behaving that are acceptable and beneficial to an individual or society. Some good habits you may already practice are as follows:

Being respectful to others

Respecting the environment

Attending school regularly

Completing assigned tasks properly and on time

Being friendly to a newcomer in your neighborhood or class

Being honest in all your activities and responsibilities

Not smoking or chewing gum

Taking care of yourself with good nutrition and exercise

Bad habits are those behaviors that are annoying or unacceptable to individuals or society. Do you have any bad habits that you need to work on? Remember, the best way to break a bad habit is to drop it.

One bad habit that causes a lot of grief is gossip. Gossip can wreck marriages, ruin reputations, and cause heartaches. Before you repeat a negative story about someone, ask yourself: Is it true? Is it fair? Is it necessary?

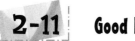 **Good Habits**

List three *good* habits you want to develop.

_____

_____

_____

2-12 Case Study

John was a new health care professional in the office. During his orientation, he presented a know-it-all attitude with his coworkers who were attempting to help him become comfortable in his new position. He was very aggressive (not assertive) and in a loud and sarcastic voice pointed out all the things wrong in the office. In addition, he went on about where he had worked before and how they had done everything right. Although his coworkers pressed him for specific examples for improvement, he really did not have any. He was appropriately told about his attitude and the potential for problems if it continued. Within 3 months, he left the job because "he could not get along with coworkers or patients." In addition, he made several errors with his patients.

Do you think his aggressive know-it all attitude was a cover for a very insecure individual, or do you have other possible explanations?

_____

_____

How would you characterize John's handling of constructive criticism?

_____

_____

_____

What specific attitudes does John need to develop before going on to his next position?

_____

_____

_____

Without taking the steps to change, what do you think John's future work record will demonstrate?

_____

_____

_____

2-13 Internet Activity

Using Internet search engines, try to find additional material on personal and professional characteristics for success that you can share with your fellow students. Some suggested keywords are: professionalism, self-motivation, lifelong learning, positive thinking, and positive attitudes. Write down something new to share.

_____

_____

_____

THOUGHTS TO PONDER

Young people represent 24% of our population and 100% of our future!

- Author Unknown

I hear and I forget, I see and I remember, I do and I understand.

- Chinese Proverb

CHAPTER 3

Setting Goals and Time Management

OBJECTIVES

Upon completion of this chapter, you should be able to:

- Set effective personal, educational, career, and community goals.
- Develop action plans to achieve *your* stated goals.
- Assess your time management skills.
- Develop effective time management skills.

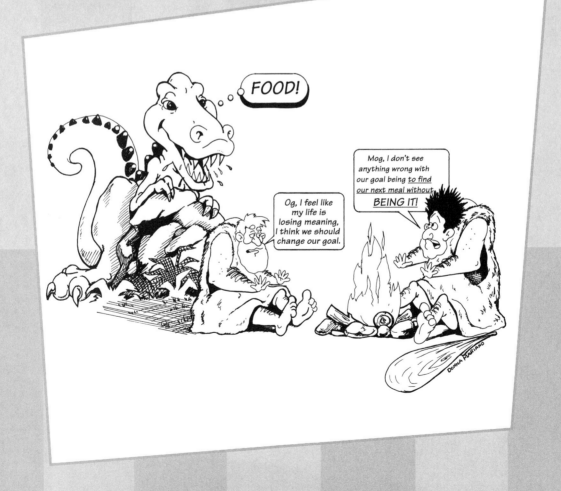

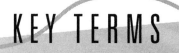

KEY TERMS

goal	objective	short-range goal
long-range goals	plateau period	time management
medium-range goal	procrastination	visualization

INTRODUCTION

Whoever wants to reach a distant goal must take many small steps.

— Helmut Schmidt

Chapter 2 gave you the opportunity to explore who you are. This chapter begins to explore where you are going and how you plan on getting there. It is important to note that people with high self-esteem not only have a positive confident attitude but also walk with a mission in mind. They are continually striving to achieve their goals or visions.

Learning to set **goals** creates the foundation for your professional image and your professional success. This chapter shows you how to set achievable goals. Although your goals may change as you mature, you should always have the goal of seeking further education and striving to better yourself.

This chapter also discusses time management. This will help you more efficiently and effectively use your time to help achieve your goals. A secondary benefit of good time management is that it will *free up* more time for you to enjoy yourself. All work and no play is not good. You must also nurture yourself and have fun. Time management will help you accomplish this task. In turn, this will make you feel better about yourself and become more committed to your goals. It all fits together.

Setting goals will be part of your everyday activity as a health care professional. You will need to develop therapeutic goals and treatment plans for your patients. In addition, in the hectic hospital environment, good time management skills are a must.

Put "the initial time" in on this chapter. Once these techniques become a part of your everyday life, it will save you a great deal of time and make you much more productive. It will also make your life much more enjoyable.

SETTING GOALS

Developing goals will help you decide where you want to go. But what are goals? Goals are specific accomplishments you aim to achieve. Effective goals should have five major characteristics as shown in Figure 3–1. Effective goals should be:

- Self-chosen
- Measurable
- Moderately challenging
- Attainable
- Positive

SELF-CHOSEN

There may be several well-meaning people in your life who might try to set goals for you. Although you should listen to them, you must ultimately choose your own goals. This gives you ownership and responsibility for your goals. Your goals should be something *you* desire and really want to do. Have you ever heard stories of patients who "willed" themselves to die? Even though the health care professional's goal was to treat them and make them better, this was not the patient's self-chosen goal.

MEASURABLE

Your goal must be specific and measurable. For example, let us say that your goal is to "do well in your health sciences courses." This is

FIGURE 3-1
Goals—the foundation upon which to live your life

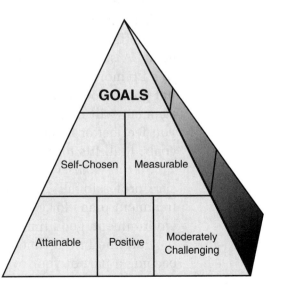

too vague. How well is well? If you state that your goal is to "get a B or better in each of your health sciences courses," you now have a measure of your success. You will know for sure if you have achieved the goal or not.

MODERATELY CHALLENGING

For example, in sports it may be easy to play against weak competition and make yourself look really good. However, you will not get better until you play against strong competition and challenge yourself to improve. Many coaches will tell you "you are only as good as your competition." In health care, you must constantly challenge yourself to learn new techniques in order to give your patients the most current and best treatments.

ATTAINABLE

You must be able to see yourself (conceive of) accomplishing this goal. You must be able to believe you can do it. Remember, if you conceive it and believe it, you can achieve it.

POSITIVE

Always use positive language when stating a goal. One goal that a group of nurses developed was to increase physician interaction. However, this can mean more conflicts between physicians and nurses. This would satisfy the goal as stated. The new goal should then become "to increase positive physician interactions."

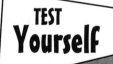

Which Is a Better Goal?

Choose the better goal statement.
1. a. I will do better with my patients and try to be more helpful.
   b. I will assess my patient interaction skills and develop action plans to improve them.
2. a. I will exercise three times a week.
   b. I will get in better shape so that I look better at the beach.
3. a. I will successfully pass the cardiopulmonary resuscitation (CPR) course.
   b. I may take a CPR course, if it is not too hard.
4. a. I will do volunteer work with senior citizens to improve my skills with geriatric patients.
   b. I will try to get to know older people better.
5. a. I will change my eating habits to maintain a weight of 150 lbs.
   b. I will not eat junk food.

OBJECTIVES

Objectives are related to goals. Objectives are things you need to do in order to achieve your stated goal. Objectives can also be thought of as the specific steps in your overall action plan to realize your goal. Developing specific objectives and action plans will ensure that you reach your goal.

For example, your goal may be to become a physical therapist who specializes in sports medicine for a professional basketball team. You must now develop an action plan comprising specific objectives that will help you reach this goal. Some of the objectives may include researching the requirements and talking to physical therapists.

TYPES OF GOALS

There are several types of goals. Goals can be broken down into specific categories to allow you to focus on the various aspects of your life. This text focuses on the following categories of goals:

- Career/professional goals
- Personal goals
- Educational goals
- Community goals

CAREER/PROFESSIONAL GOALS

These are the goals related to obtaining the career of your choice. Once you obtain your career, you can then make specific professional goals to improve your knowledge and skills so that you can be the best health care provider in your chosen health profession.

PERSONAL GOALS

You may have personal goals, such as to improve your self-esteem or a relationship with someone. You may also want to improve your physical well-being. These goals can include learning a new skill or hobby. Perhaps you want to learn to play the guitar or paint.

EDUCATIONAL GOALS

You may have educational goals such as completing this year with a B+ average. However, these are not just school-related goals. For example, a goal may be to learn a new technique such as CPR, first aid, word processing, or sign language. All of these would help complement your health professional skills.

COMMUNITY GOALS

We are all part of a community. Becoming involved in your community can help improve neighborhood conditions. In addition, it will give you valuable skills and experience and may help you make contacts that will be beneficial to your future. This is definitely a win-win situation. This means you win, or gain benefit, from this interaction, and your community wins by being improved. These goals may include volunteer work with the homeless or senior citizens. Another goal may be coaching children in your community or teaching illiterate adults to read.

It is important to achieve a balance with your types of goals. If you have all educational goals and no personal development goals, you may soon "burn out" from not taking care of yourself. Your educational goals will then suffer. So develop a balance of goals that will complement each other.

Goals can also be broken down according to the time frame in which they will be accomplished. You can have **short-**, **medium-**, or **long-range goals**.

- Short range: to be accomplished tomorrow, next week, next month
- Medium range: to be accomplished within the next 6 months or year
- Long range: to be accomplished within the next 3–5 years

Short- and medium-range goals are needed to accomplish your long-range goals, as illustrated in Figure 3–2.

USEFUL HINTS ON GOAL SETTING

One hint is to prioritize your goals so that you get a timeline of when they need to be accomplished. Remember, when changes occur you may need to reprioritize your goals or develop new objectives.

Visualization can also help you reach your goal. Visualize what it will be like when you have reached your goal. Picture and feel all the good feelings. This will help you maintain your commitment.

Many people go "gung ho" toward a goal for a while and then taper off. This is natural. At first you may make rapid progress toward a goal. Eventually, you may reach a period when this progress stalls. This is called a **plateau period**, where you see little or no progress toward your goal. This is the crucial stage in which you should not give up! Realize that everyone reaches this plateau period and that it will pass.

Finally, talk to other people who have achieved the goal you are working toward. Find out what they did. Learn from their mistakes. They may also prove to be valuable contacts in the future.

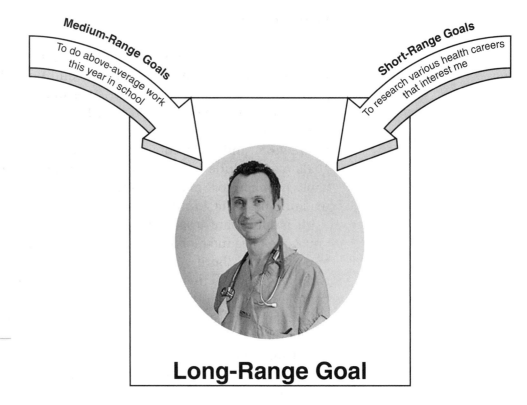

FIGURE 3-2
Obtaining long-range
goals

 What Do YOU Think?

The United States Olympic Training Program

The United States Olympic organization has developed a training program to have their athletes "think" like winners. It includes the following four main components:

- Visualize yourself in the successful performance of your event.
- Set short- and long-term goals to achieve "the gold."
- Practice physical and mental relaxation techniques.
- Concentrate on positive thoughts.

How does this relate to what you have learned so far? How does it apply to your life? What about your future health care career?

LEARNER:

Go to page 57 and complete the Critical Thinking and Application Activities 3–1, 3–2, and 3–3.

TIME MANAGEMENT

> **T**o think too long about doing a thing often becomes its undoing.
>
> - Eva Young

Someone once said that time is life. Therefore, if you waste time, you are actually wasting your life. However, be careful not to take this view too far. Taking a walk in the woods may be considered by some to be a waste of time, but it is not. Taking that walk may give you time to clear your mind, recharge your batteries, or just enjoy the beauty of nature. This certainly is time well spent. However, balance is the key. If you always walk in the woods and do not do the things you need to do in your life, it can have serious consequences.

It is best to think of time as an unrenewable resource. Therefore, use it wisely. You may have heard of the saying "carpe diem," which is Latin for seize the day. But to truly be an effective time manager and to live life to its fullest, you should "seize the moment."

TEST Yourself

Do You Need to Be a Better Time Manager?

Check the following items that relate to you.

1. _____ I complain about lack of time or say there is not enough time in the day.
2. _____ I put things off till the last minute.
3. _____ I get stressed out when given a large assignment.
4. _____ Deadlines make me anxious.
5. _____ I am often late for appointments or turning in assignments.
6. _____ I get overwhelmed with a task and do not know where to start.
7. _____ I talk for long periods on the telephone.
8. _____ I jump from one task to another.

If you checked one or two items, you are a good time manager and can work on only those areas. If you checked three or four items, you are fair and could use some help. If you checked five or six, you are a poor time manager and would greatly benefit from this chapter. If you checked seven or eight, it means that if you follow through with the suggestions and work in this chapter, it will be a positive life-changing experience.

USING TIME MANAGEMENT TECHNIQUES

Where do you start? The good news is that you have already started. Establishing goals and priorities is the first and best place to start. Goals tell us what is important and the priorities help us focus our energy on the more urgent issues.

Now that you have goals and priorities established, you can assess your time use. You can then develop plans and use tools and techniques to optimize your **time management skills**. Figure 3–3 shows the relationship between goals and time management.

To become an effective time manager, you must look at three areas:

- Minimize the "time wasters" in your life.
- Make effective lists.
- Capitalize on your personal peak periods of productivity.

MINIMIZE TIME WASTERS

Have you ever heard someone say "there aren't enough hours in the day"? Well, the truth is everyone has 24 hours in a day. If you know of a place that has more, many people will want to move there. Seriously, we all have the same amount of time. How we use our time is what makes the difference. One of the first assessment techniques is to identify "common time wasters" that could free up valuable time for other pursuits. On the following two pages is a list of common time wasters.

Failure to Plan and Establish Priorities. Without a plan, you have no sense of direction and can wander aimlessly. This wastes time.

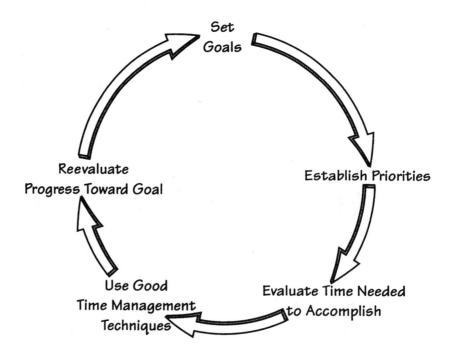

FIGURE 3-3
The whole picture: how goals and effective time management are integrated

You may say, "Yeah, but it takes time to plan!" This is certainly true, but the small amount of time invested in the plan can free up the tremendous amount of time you would waste without it. Part of the plan has to include priorities. You will be working on this soon, but let me give you one example.

Say you had six patients to do therapies on during morning rounds, which last from 7:30 to 9:30 AM. Each therapy takes about 15 minutes, and breakfast trays come at 0800. You cannot do therapies while the patients are eating. Four of your patients are fresh postoperative patients and have nasogastric tubes inserted. This means that they cannot eat. How would you plan and prioritize your morning rounds to give all the patients an effective and timely treatment?

Overplanning and Overorganizing. You can take planning and organizing to the extreme. Again, come back to the very important point that *you must find a balance.* If you put so much time into developing and organizing a plan, you will have little time for doing anything else.

The Telephone/Cell Phones. The telephone is one of the most useful facilitators of communication ever invented. However, many people can let this device completely control their lives and waste a lot of time. I am not saying that talking to your friends is a waste of time. This is important, but again you must strike a balance. To call someone you have just seen in school and gossip for hours certainly is not a productive use of time. Using the telephone for personal matters during work hours has been identified as a major reason for low productivity in health care.

The Computer. While the computer is a great time-saving device in many applications such as researching topics and writing reports, it can become a time waster if abused. For example, one can spend too much time in chat rooms, tied up with e-mail and instant messages, or playing computer games and not have enough time to get one's academic and clinical work done. One should enjoy the computer, but again maintaining balance is the key.

Personal Habits. Two personal habits that are huge wasters of time are **procrastination** and worry. Procrastination is putting things off until the last minute. Procrastination can be caused by lack of priorities, boredom, anxiety, or fear of failure. It can also be caused by being uncertain about what the task is.

Procrastination and worry are related. Procrastination robs you of time and power by causing stress in the form of guilt, embarrassment, and anxiety. The anxiety and fear of failure can cause worry. Worry is such a powerful enemy of time and causes great stresses on the mind and body that a portion of the next chapter is devoted to it. For now, consider the following: *Many people worry so much about failing that they never accomplish what it was they were worried about.*

Do not procrastinate any longer. Take a look at the list that shows you ways to combat time wasters. And as the famous commercial says, "Just Do It."

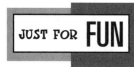

Prioritizing Tasks

Let's say you have reached your long-range career goal and are now a hospital staff member (soon to be promoted) working the daylight, or 7 to 3, shift. You have the following tasks to do. Prioritize this list by writing numbers 1 to 10 on the line to the left of the item, indicating which you would do first, second, and so on. The hospital works on military time, so you might have to review or research how that works. It is very simple.

_____ Do afternoon treatment rounds (1300 to 1430).

_____ Research at the library for a report to your medical director due in 2 weeks.

_____ Reserve a conference room for an in-service for your department. This must be done by 1100.

_____ Do morning treatment rounds (0715 to 0915).

_____ Call two home care patients to reschedule appointments for tomorrow.

_____ Fix and calibrate equipment in the utility room. This will take about 1 hour.

_____ Complete billing charges for yesterday—must be done by end of shift and will take about 30 minutes.

_____ Eat lunch with medical equipment salesperson.

_____ Give end-of-shift report to oncoming 3 to 11 shift (about 30 minutes).

_____ Scheduled meeting from 0930 to 1000 with department director concerning my up-coming promotion and raise for doing such a professional job.

COMBATING TIME WASTERS: PROCRASTINATION AND WORRY

- Of course, *organize* and *plan.*
- If you are uncertain of what needs to be done, ask!
- Set your priorities so that you are not jumping from one task to another.
- Find ways of making the job interesting. Have fun with what you are doing. Be happy and have a positive attitude.
- Do your most demanding work when you are fresh and alert.
- Reward yourself when you get a job done.
- Organize your desk so that you are not wasting time trying to find pencils, dictionaries, and so on.
- Make use of "found time" such as waiting in lines or at the doctor's office.

- Take care of yourself! Go to bed a little earlier to recharge your batteries. Get up a half hour sooner to gain productive time. The morning is usually your best and most productive time.
- Control interruptions when doing a task. These can include phone calls and visitors.
- Finish what you start.

MAKING EFFECTIVE LISTS

Many successful health care leaders state "making lists" is the secret of their success. This allows them to plan and prioritize their tasks. It also helps them generate ideas and see better ways of combining tasks.

There are several types of lists you can make and several places you can make them. The process of keeping different types of lists can become so confusing that you can become lost in all your lists. Therefore, I recommend a somewhat simpler way to organize your life. The first step is to get the proper tools to help you.

The most important tool is a large desk calendar for your special study area, Figure 3–4. This can allow you to put all your special up-coming events and deadlines in one place, and at a glance, you can see what your future holds. This type of planning gives you an overview or the entire picture. You can carry a pocket planner with you to mark down things as they come up during the day and then transfer them to your desk calendar.

In the electronic age, handheld computers can help you to maintain daily schedules and even produce a calendar of obligations. However, it is important to have something in front of you that shows the "big picture." A store-bought desk calendar or an electronically produced one that you print out facilitates seeing everything at a glance and helps in strategic planning.

| Notes: | | | | | | |
Sunday	Monday	Tuesday	Wednesday	Thursday	Friday	Saturday
		1 Think of possible topics	2	3 Choose paper topic and title	4	5 Library research— 2.5 hours
6 Library research— 2.5 hours	7 Mom's Birthday	8 Library research— 2.5 hours	9 Dance class 4:00 p.m.	10	11 Library research— 2.5 hours	12 Develop outline
13	14 Finish outline	15	16	17 Write rough draft	18	19
20	21 Finish rough draft	22	23 Dance class 4:00 p.m.	24 Rewrite final paper	25	26
27	28 Turn in paper	29	30 PAPER DUE!!!			

September 2006

FIGURE 3-4
Example of a large desk calendar

Now you need to develop more specific plans to meet your deadlines and fulfill your obligations. Pick the major tasks along with their deadlines that are coming up within the next month or so. Now brainstorm and plan all the activities needed to complete the tasks within the deadline. For example, you may have a research paper due in 4 weeks. You would break the task into a logical sequence of events with an approximate time needed to complete each step. This may include the following:

1. Choosing a topic and title (1 or 2 days to think about)
2. Researching and gathering information (10 hours at library)
3. Developing an outline (12 hours)
4. Writing a rough draft (16 hours)
5. Rewriting final paper (6 hours)

You can see from your calendar where you have the time to fill in for each of these tasks. Make sure you give yourself plenty of time before the deadline to have your paper completed. This will provide a buffer zone in case you underestimated the time needed for a certain task or if something unexpected comes up. You can write these tasks on your desk calendar in blocks of time. For example, you might break your library time into 4 days of 2.5 hours each. Remember, your first couple of attempts are learning experiences. Keep records so that you can improve. Now that you have your major tasks planned, you can continue to update your calendar and repeat this process with each new assignment.

The Daily To-Do List. Now you need to move on to a very important list, your daily to-do list. This should be done at your special study area with your calendar in front of you. A daily to-do list can be your most effective tool when referenced to your desk calendar. To construct this list, do the following:

1. Write down every activity, assignment, meeting, or promise that comes your way each day.
2. Do what activities you can as they occur, if time permits.
3. At the end of your day, prioritize your list. Place at top the tasks that need done the next day and mark them with an asterisk. Then list other tasks that would be nice to do and may even get you ahead. Remember to check your desk calendar for the next day when making this list. Now go to bed, secure in the knowledge that you do not have to worry about the next day.
4. Consult your list during the day, and cross off any task when completed. Crossing off the task should give you a sense of accomplishment. You should really derive pleasure from crossing off items on your list. This will reinforce your good behavior and keep you dedicated to your list. You should have all top-priority items crossed off at the end of the day.

5. Now make a new list for the next day. Get in the habit of spending a few minutes each day planning for the following day. It will help you greatly. This process will eventually become automatic.

CAPITALIZE ON PEAK PERIODS

> **W**hy is it I get my best ideas during the morning while I'm shaving?
>
> - Albert Einstein

During the study skills section, you assessed whether you were a morning or evening person. Most people are most productive in the morning, but we all differ. Know what times of day are most productive for you, and schedule your more difficult tasks for these times.

You will also notice that your patients will also have peak periods when they respond to therapies better. In addition, they will have periods of distress, usually occurring at night. Have you ever noticed how you may feel sicker or more anxious at night?

Even seasonal changes can alter your productivity or feeling of well-being. Health studies show that depression and illness rise in areas where there is less sunlight. That is why a bright and cheery room in the dark of winter can be good medicine.

WORDS TO THE WISE

You have done a great job planning. However, life rarely goes as planned. This is why you must be flexible and positive. If something unexpected comes up, do not panic or get negative and worry. This accomplishes nothing. Calm down, reorganize, and do what you can do.

Also know when you are overcommitted, and learn to say no. Remember, do not be a slave to your schedule or your lists. You do not have to make large lists. Make sure they are reasonable and give you time for yourself during the day.

Periodically reward yourself for getting all your tasks done. If you have a large task (e.g., that research paper), reward yourself along the way for each little step accomplished. This will help your motivation. But remember to save the biggest reward for when your large task is done.

SUMMARY

Setting goals and using good time management techniques are the tools you can use for your personal and professional success. Your goals should be self-chosen, measurable, moderately challenging, attainable, and positive. They should include both personal and professional types of goals. Time management techniques will help you to effectively and efficiently reach your goals. These techniques should include an assessment of time wasters in your life, using effective lists, and capitalizing on your personal periods of peak productivity.

LEARNER:

Go to page 63 and complete the Critical Thinking and Application Activities 3–4, 3–5, 3–6, 3–7, and 3–8.

Why These Activities Are Important to You

Learning how to set proper goals will give you your vision and direction in life. How many people do you know who say they are lost or have no direction in life? Many of them lack goals. But goals alone will not make everything all right. You need to know and practice the skills needed to obtain your goals.

One major skill is effective time management. You may need to invest some time initially to learn these skills, but they will pay off in a big way. They will bring a sense of order and focus to your life. These skills will also help you free up time to enjoy yourself and recharge your energy.

CRITICAL THINKING AND APPLICATION ACTIVITIES

3-1   Developing Long-Range Goals

This chapter states that goals should be:

- Self-chosen
- Measurable
- Moderately challenging
- Attainable
- Positive

Use these criteria to develop a long-range (within 5 years) goal for each of the four types of goals discussed in your text.

Example:

Type of goal: *career/professional—long range*

Range and date of accomplishment: *within 5 years*

Your goal: *to graduate with an associate degree from an accredited respiratory therapy school. I will graduate in the top 10 percent of my class.*

Reason you chose this goal: *I had severe asthma as a child and realize the importance of being able to breathe. I want to make a difference in patients who are fighting for each breath.*

Type of goal: *career/professional—long range*

Range and date of accomplishment: *within 5 years*

Your goal: _____

_____

Reason you chose this goal: _____

_____

Now compare your goal to the criteria list. Check off each criterion and rewrite your statement if needed until you have included all the criteria.

1. _____ Self-chosen
2. _____ Measurable
3. _____ Moderately challenging
4. _____ Attainable
5. _____ Positive

Type of goal: *personal—long range*

Range and date of accomplishment: *within 5 years*

Your goal: _____

_____

Reason you chose this goal: _____

_____

Now compare your goal to the criteria list. Check off each criterion and rewrite your statement if needed until you have included all the criteria.

1. _____ Self-chosen
2. _____ Measurable
3. _____ Moderately challenging
4. _____ Attainable
5. _____ Positive

Type of goal: *educational—long range*
Range and date of accomplishment: *within 5 years*
Your goal: _____

_____

Reason you chose this goal: _____

_____

Now compare your goal to the criteria list. Check off each criterion and rewrite your statement if needed until you have included all the criteria.

1. _____ Self-chosen
2. _____ Measurable
3. _____ Moderately challenging
4. _____ Attainable
5. _____ Positive

Type of goal: *community—long range*
Range and date of accomplishment: *within 5 years*
Your goal: _____

_____

Reason you chose this goal: _____

_____

Now compare your goal to the criteria list. Check off each criterion and rewrite your statement if needed until you have included all the criteria.

1. _____ Self-chosen
2. _____ Measurable
3. _____ Moderately challenging
4. _____ Attainable
5. _____ Positive

3-2 Refining Your Long-Range Goals

Now, rewrite each of the previous goals to include an action plan that contains specific objectives and resources that will help you in your quest.

Example:

Type of goal: *career/professional—long range*
Range and date of accomplishment: *within 5 years*

Your goal: *to graduate with an associate degree from an accredited respiratory therapy school. I will graduate in the top 10 percent of my class.*

Reason you chose this goal: *I had severe asthma as a child and realize the importance of being able to breathe. I want to make a difference in patients who are fighting for each breath.*

Action plan (specific objectives):

1. *Investigate the field of respiratory care and determine requirements.*
2. *Do "B" work or better in my health science courses to get accepted to the program.*
3. *Do volunteer work and get to know some future contacts within the profession.*

Resources to help achieve: *my health science teachers, local hospital, library, local community college and my determination to succeed*

YOUR GOALS AND ACTION PLANS

Type of goal: _____

Range and date of accomplishment: _____

Your goal: _____

_____

Reason you chose this goal: _____

_____

Action plan (specific objectives):

1. _____
2. _____
3. _____

Resources to help achieve it: _____

_____

Type of goal: _____

Range and date of accomplishment: _____

Your goal: _____

_____

Reason you chose this goal: _____

_____

Action plan (specific objectives):

1. _____
2. _____
3. _____

Resources to help achieve it: _____

_____

Type of goal: _____

Range and date of accomplishment: _____

Your goal: _____

_____

Reason you chose this goal: _____

_____

Action plan (specific objectives):

  1. _____

  2. _____

  3. _____

Resources to help achieve it: _____

_____

Type of goal: _____

Range and date of accomplishment: _____

Your goal: _____

_____

Reason you chose this goal: _____

_____

Action plan (specific objectives):

  1. _____

  2. _____

  3. _____

Resources to help achieve it: _____

_____

 3-3 ## Developing Short- and Medium-Range Goals

Now that you have completed your long-term goals, you have your vision. You are not going to achieve this overnight. You must now take small steps in your journey. You must develop short- and medium-range goals to achieve your long-range goals. For each of your long-range goals, write one short-term (within a month) and write one medium-term (accomplished within 6 months) goal that will complement your long-range goal and move you toward it.

Type of goal: _____

Range and date of accomplishment: _____

Your goal: _____

_____

Reason you chose this goal: _____

_____

Action plan (specific objectives):

  1. _____

  2. _____

  3. _____

Resources to help achieve it: _____

_____

Type of goal: _____

Range and date of accomplishment: _____

Your goal: _____
_____

Reason you chose this goal: _____
_____

Action plan (specific objectives):

   1. _____

   2. _____

   3. _____

Resources to help achieve it: _____
_____

Type of goal: _____

Range and date of accomplishment: _____

Your goal: _____
_____

Reason you chose this goal: _____
_____

Action plan (specific objectives):

   1. _____

   2. _____

   3. _____

Resources to help achieve it: _____
_____

Type of goal: _____

Range and date of accomplishment: _____

Your goal: _____
_____

Reason you chose this goal: _____
_____

Action plan (specific objectives):

   1. _____

   2. _____

   3. _____

Resources to help achieve it: _____
_____

Type of goal: _____

Range and date of accomplishment: _____

Your goal: _____

_____

Reason you chose this goal: _____

_____

Action plan (specific objectives):

   1. _____

   2. _____

   3. _____

Resources to help achieve it: _____

_____

Type of goal: _____

Range and date of accomplishment: _____

Your goal: _____

_____

Reason you chose this goal: _____

_____

Action plan (specific objectives):

   1. _____

   2. _____

   3. _____

Resources to help achieve it: _____

_____

Type of goal: _____

Range and date of accomplishment: _____

Your goal: _____

_____

Reason you chose this goal: _____

_____

Action plan (specific objectives):

   1. _____

   2. _____

   3. _____

Resources to help achieve it: _____

_____

Type of goal: _____

Range and date of accomplishment: _____

Your goal: _____

_____

Reason you chose this goal: _____

_____

Action plan (specific objectives):

  1. _____

  2. _____

  3. _____

Resources to help achieve it: _____

_____

3-4   Identifying Time Wasters

Good, effective time management will help you meet deadlines, help you perform better academically, and give you more *free* time. The first step in becoming a good time manager is to identify your time wasters.

    Review the list of time wasters in your book. Recopy them here. For 1 week, put a check mark next to each time waster you performed. At the end of the week, see which ones have the most "checks" beside them. Now develop your own goal and action plan to combat your worst time waster habit.

_____

_____

_____

_____

_____

_____

_____

_____

_____

_____

_____

_____

_____

3-5   Working with Your Calendar

If you do not already have one, obtain a large desk calendar and fill in all your commitments, social activities, assignment deadlines, sports activities, and scheduled workdays. Keep it neat. Now take one of your academic deadlines or projects and break it down into manageable steps with approximate times for completion.

List these here and then return to your calendar and place the steps in the appropriate gaps. Make sure you are scheduled to complete the project ahead of your deadline.

Project: _____

Steps: _____

_____

_____

_____

_____

3-6   Making a Daily To-Do List

a. Make a list of all tasks you want to accomplish tomorrow. Assign a priority by placing an asterisk or star next to the tasks that cannot be delayed and must be done tomorrow.

b. Place a number 1 by the tasks that are important and need to be done as soon as possible.

c. Place a number 2 next to the tasks that can be delayed for a while but, if time permits, could get you ahead of schedule. Limit yourself to only a few number 1 and 2 tasks.

d. Do this in consultation with your desk calendar for 7 consecutive days. Then evaluate your performance and learn how you can improve on your list-making skills and incorporate this process into your life.

Hint: Keep your lists short and simple as possible—do not try to do everything in one day. Remember to cross off items when done. I purposely did not put a column for you to check off when each task is done. You can derive more pleasure and sense of accomplishment from crossing out the entire task.

Example:

THINGS TO DO TODAY LIST   DATE: 11-5-05

Priority	Task
*	*Finish anatomy and physiology questions due 11/6.*
2	*Do library research for paper due Jan. 10.*
1	*Clean my room and organize my study area and closet.*
1	*Call the hospital to set up volunteer work for next week.*
*	*Get essential groceries for Grandma.*
*	*Soccer game at 6 PM.*
2	*Come up with an idea for science project, due Jan. 20.*
*	*Return Joshua's CPR manual, which he lent me last week.*

Your List

THINGS TO DO TODAY LIST   DATE _____

Priority	Task
_____	_____
_____	_____
_____	_____
_____	_____
_____	_____
_____	_____
_____	_____

THINGS TO DO TODAY LIST   DATE _____

Priority   **Task**

_____   _____
_____   _____
_____   _____
_____   _____
_____   _____
_____   _____
_____   _____
_____   _____

THINGS TO DO TODAY LIST   DATE _____

Priority   **Task**

_____   _____
_____   _____
_____   _____
_____   _____
_____   _____
_____   _____
_____   _____
_____   _____

THINGS TO DO TODAY LIST   DATE _____

Priority   **Task**

_____   _____
_____   _____
_____   _____
_____   _____
_____   _____
_____   _____
_____   _____
_____   _____

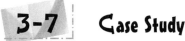 ## Case Study

Mary had a difficult time in her health care training and barely managed to graduate. She decided to try goal setting when she got hired in her first new job. She made only one goal, and it was as follows: "I want to be the department director within a year." After her first year Mary was not the department director and was very frustrated with her position and felt that goal setting was a bunch of "hogwash" and really doesn't work.

Did Mary really understand the goal-setting process? What were the mistakes she made and how could she correct them?

_____
_____
_____
_____

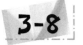 **Internet Activity**

Using Internet search engines, try to find additional material on goal setting and time management that can help you and your fellow students. Some suggested keywords are: goal setting, time management techniques, preventing procrastination, avoiding worry, and achieving goals. Write down something new that you found to share.

_____

_____

_____

THOUGHTS TO PONDER

1. Your goals can be changed.
2. Reward yourself when you reach short- and medium-range goals. This will reenergize you and give you a sense of movement and accomplishment toward your long-range goals.
3. You can make several more short- and medium-range goals. However, do not make many more long-range goals than one or two per category or you may get overwhelmed.
4. Place your completed long-range goals in a prominent area in your portfolio and post a copy in your study area. This will keep them in your mind.

Congratulations, you now have good long-range goals established and one of the major tools (time management) to help you get there. Keep up the good work!

CHAPTER 4

Stress Management

OBJECTIVES

Upon completion of this chapter, you should be able to:

- Identify the different types of stress and their effects on your mind and body.
- Use the three-point system to effectively manage stress in your life.
- Learn physical and emotional coping techniques to deal with stress.

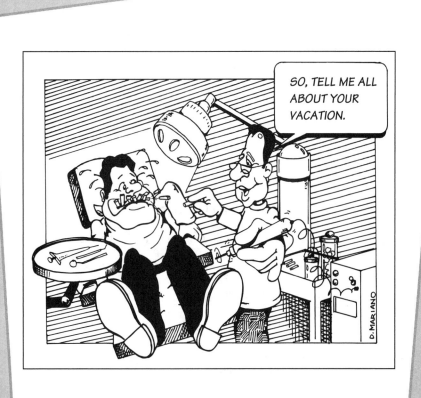

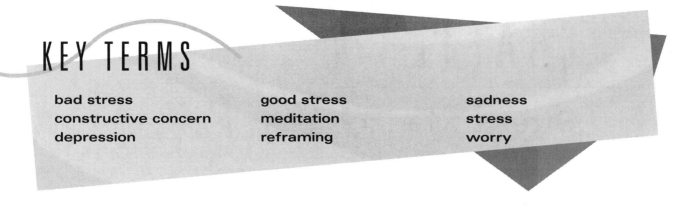

KEY TERMS

bad stress

constructive concern

depression

good stress

meditation

reframing

sadness

stress

worry

INTRODUCTION

You now have your goals and vision of the future along with effective time management techniques to help you on your journey. Along the way toward your goals, stress will be something you will have to contend with. When you reach your goal as a health care practitioner, the stress will not end. Watch any good television show or read any novel about a hospital and you will see many situations that can be stressful. For example, one of the more common medical abbreviations used in the hospital is *stat,* which means right away, or as we jokingly say, you should have been there and done it by now.

As a future health care professional, you must know how to care for yourself first before you can effectively care for others. This means that you need to learn about stress, how to cope with stress, and how to use stress to your advantage. Stress can be a powerful motivator for growth. However, if you do not learn to control it, stress can control your life and take a terrible toll. Remember, without you, there will not be someone there to make the difference in a patient's recovery.

What Do YOU Think?

Stress in Health Care

What types of stress do you think you'll encounter in the hospital? What about dealing with patients or their families?

How will you handle your first patient's death?

What if you make a mistake in treating a patient?

These questions should cause you to think and probably will cause some stress. Feeling some stress is good and normal. Stress can help you grow and prepare for what lies ahead. The good news is that you can learn to use stress to your advantage. Learning how to deal with stress will allow you to have a much fuller and more rewarding life. Making stress your friend will prepare you for the wonderful challenges life has to offer.

UNDERSTANDING STRESS

To be able to conquer and harness stress to your advantage, you must first understand what stress is all about. It is important to realize that no situation or event by itself causes us stress. Rather it is how we "perceive" a situation that causes stress. It is our internal response to external stimuli.

For example, two individuals may receive an injection. They will both undergo the *same* procedure with the *same* technician in the *same* environment. One individual may not feel any stress or anxiety, whereas the other may be highly stressed at the thought of getting a shot, as in Figure 4–1. Therefore stress, like beauty, is in the eye of the beholder. Stress occurs as a result of how we interpret and react to a situation or event. It can be positive or negative, major or minor.

Stress can have many definitions. For now, we will define stress as how our mind and body react to an environment that is largely shaped by our perceptions of an event or situation. Now that we have defined stress, let us take a closer look at the different types of stress and the physical and psychological reactions that can occur.

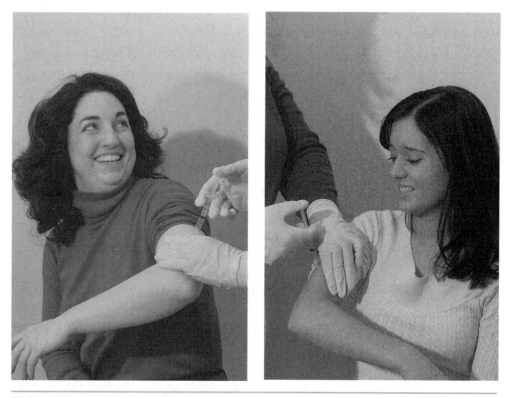

FIGURE 4-1
Different reactions to the same event. Who perceives stress?

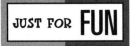

There are many common expressions that relate to stress. Some examples include the following:

I was so scared I lost my breath.

I was breathless with excitement. (Remember stress can be good.)

I can now breathe easier.

My heart was pounding.

My brain is fried.

My stomach was twisted in knots.

Notice how these relate stress to physiologic activities. The mind and body are truly related. What implications can this have for your patients? Can you think of other statements?

TYPES OF STRESS AND ITS EFFECTS

The first time you are called on to perform cardiopulmonary resuscitation (CPR) on an arrest victim is probably going to be a stressful event in your life. Even though you practiced and trained hard, you are still uncertain of how it will be in a real life-and-death situation. This is normal. Your physical and psychological symptoms may include the following:

- Increased adrenaline levels for more energy
- Faster heart rate (tachycardia) to supply more oxygen to muscles
- Increased blood pressure to get more blood flow to the brain
- Pupil dilation to bring in more light
- Faster breathing (tachypnea) to bring in more oxygen
- Heightened state of awareness to focus on the job at hand
- Mild level of anxiety to keep you sharp and not take the situation too lightly

These can all be helpful reactions that enhance your performance. Therefore, you can have **good stress** and **bad stress**. The key again is balance or moderation. Figure 4–2 graphically illustrates good versus bad stress. A little stress will get you "up" for the task at hand. However, if you let stress get out of hand and panic, you now have bad stress and your anxiety level rises to the point where you perform poorly or even not at all.

Hans Seyle, the father of stress research, coined the term eustress to describe positive stress. "Eu" means good or well. Seyle used the term distress for negative stress. This worktext will simply use the terms good and bad stress to help to personalize the terms in your life.

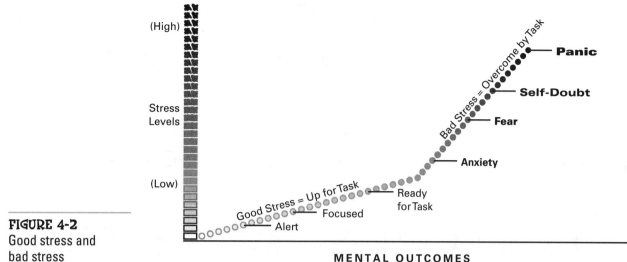

FIGURE 4-2
Good stress and
bad stress

Both positive and negative experiences can cause stress. For example, if your first CPR experience was successful it will cause less stress than a negative experience. The mere fact that this is your "first" real CPR experience makes it stressful because the experience is unpredictable or unknown. Afterward, you will have gained experience. Even if you made mistakes, you will learn from those mistakes and know what to expect the next time. Therefore, unpredictable events are more stressful than predictable events.

Stress can also relate to time. We all have temporary stressors (factors that cause stress) in our lives. However, when a stressor becomes constant, it has serious effects on our body and mind. Continual or constant stress can lead to the following:

- High blood pressure, heart attack, or stroke
- Stomach ulcers
- Lack of sleep or insomnia
- Decreased immune system functioning
- Depression and personality changes

Temporary controlled stress can help us perform better. Indeed, any time you try something new or meet a new challenge, stress can be a powerful friend. This is how we grow and develop. Continual uncontrolled stress will exact a price on our minds and bodies. Figure 4–3 contrasts good versus bad stress. Trying to maintain balance and control over stress is discussed shortly.

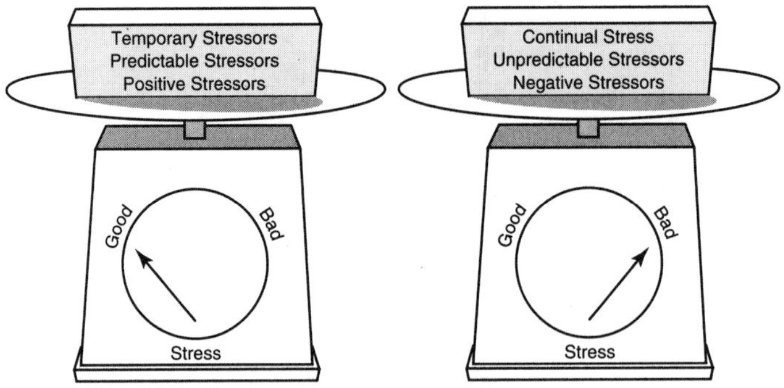

FIGURE 4-3
Types of stressors

TEST Yourself

Do You Need This Chapter?

Rate the following statements with numbers 1 through 4 as follows:

1. Never   2. Sometimes   3. Often   4. Always

1. _____ I feel tired.
2. _____ I worry a lot about problems or how things are going to turn out.
3. _____ I can spot all the things others are doing wrong.
4. _____ I need to be perfect at what I do.
5. _____ I do very little exercise.
6. _____ I feel sad.
7. _____ I am very competitive and need to win to feel good about myself.
8. _____ I take on everyone else's problems
9. _____ I try to control others.
10. _____ I cannot do anything right.
11. _____ I avoid risks for fear of failure.
12. _____ I let my work pile up.
13. _____ I feel like I'm being pulled in all directions.
14. _____ I have a very negative attitude.
15. _____ I get headaches.
16. _____ I have too much to do and too little time to do it.
17. _____ I overreact to situations.
18. _____ I feel guilty if I relax and do nothing.
19. _____ I talk very quickly.
20. _____ I get angry easily.

Total Points _____

Now use your total to see where you stand:

Over 60–80   This chapter could be a life-changing experience.

50–59   You desperately need to work on this chapter.

40–49   You would gain moderate benefit from this chapter.

30–39   You are doing pretty good but can improve slightly.

20–29   Maybe you should write a book on handling stress.

LEARNER:

Go to page 83 and complete the Critical Thinking and Application Activity 4–1.

A SIMPLIFIED STRESS MANAGEMENT SYSTEM

There are several systems of stress management. I believe the simplest and most logical is to break down stress management into the following three areas:

- Recognize your stress signals and stress producers.

- Be concerned but avoid worrying!

- Develop coping strategies.

First, recognizing your own stressors and the symptoms they cause can help you determine when your stress is out of balance. These signals can be valuable to your good health and positive attitude. They represent a "wake-up call" that says you need to cope with what is going on in your life before it overtakes you.

Second, remove **worry** from your life. Worry is wasted negative energy. If you can learn to stop worrying (and you can), you will gain back energy to grow.

Finally, part of the stress management system is developing effective coping mechanisms to deal with and minimize the negative stressors in your life. These are not only very effective, but also very fun if approached with a positive attitude. See Figure 4–4.

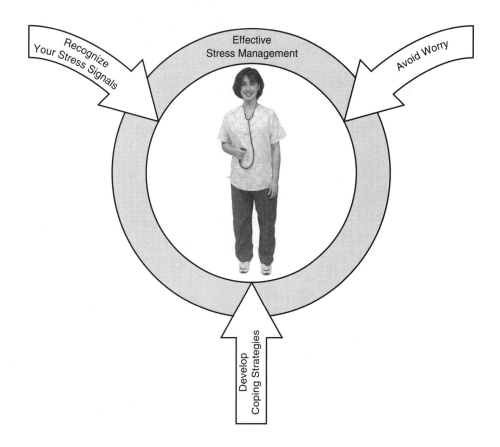

FIGURE 4-4
Three-point stress
management system

RECOGNIZING YOUR STRESS SIGNALS

As already stated, a certain amount of stress is normal. We need it to develop and grow. However, going beyond minimal stress levels for sustained periods can be harmful. You need to determine when you are losing balance. The best way is to look for signs or indicators that the stress is too much. Table 4–1 shows the physical changes and emotional changes that signal too much stress.

It is important to differentiate **depression** from **sadness**. If someone is sad after a painful disappointment or the loss of a loved one, this is a normal part of the grieving process. However, if the sadness remains for a prolonged period and interferes with the ability to go about your daily business, it becomes depression. Again, moderation is the key.

Looking at the list of stress signs should paint a pretty good visual picture of what high levels of stress can cause. It is no wonder that individuals who cannot handle stress have more accidents, have poorer attendance, and are unable to study and learn. It also means they have poorer relationships and difficulty interacting with others. Besides, who would want to constantly feel like the picture the list describes? Do you think this would be the kind of health care professional you would want to treat you?

TABLE 4-1
The Physical and Emotional Signs of Stress

PHYSICAL CHANGES	EMOTIONAL CHANGES
Headaches	Lack of concentration
Shortness of breath	Irritability
Increased pulse rate	Anger
Nausea	Mood swings
Insomnia	Overreactiveness
Fatigue	Depression
Neck or back pain	Eating disorders
Dermatological problems	Anxiety
Chronic constipation/diarrhea	Low self-image
	Hopeless feelings

TEST Yourself

How Many Stress Signals Do You Have?

How many of the following signals do you have on a regular basis (once or twice every week)? If you checked two or fewer signals, you are doing pretty good and need minor improvement. If you checked three or more, you need to work hard on how you are handling stress.

1. _____ Headaches
2. _____ Shortness of breath
3. _____ Fast or irregular pulse
4. _____ Nausea
5. _____ Insomnia
6. _____ Difficulty eating
7. _____ Sadness
8. _____ Chronic fatigue
9. _____ Irritability
10. _____ Hostility
11. _____ Mood swings
12. _____ Feelings of being overwhelmed
13. _____ Difficulty concentrating
14. _____ Neck or back pain
15. _____ Chronic diarrhea

RECOGNIZING YOUR STRESS PRODUCERS

Everyone has stress signals that tell them when they need to slow down and reevaluate their stress management. When these signals occur, sit back and try to identify what is causing this extra stress so that you can then effectively cope. The following list represents some common stress producers that can quickly get out of hand. This by no means is a complete list, but it represents some of the more common excessive stress producers.

- Self-doubts or lack of confidence in our abilities
- Lack of personal organization
- Inability to plan or prioritize work
- Perfectionism
- Placement of excessive demands on ourselves
- Inability to say no
- Tendency to take all problems and criticisms personally
- Inflexibility and lack of openness to change

Finally, negative thinking or thought patterns can add excessive stress to our lives. People who are in the habit of thinking in negative ways feel out of control. They think thoughts such as "I'll never learn this technique" or "My patients will never like me." All these thoughts are sending a message that "You are helpless and 'never' will accomplish your goal." You have already set up a negative self-fulfilling prophecy. The computer programmers have a saying "GIGO," which stands for garbage in, garbage out. Do you see how this can relate to negative thinking or programming?

Go to page 83 and complete the Critical Thinking and Application Activities 4–2 and 4–3.

WORRY, WORRY, WORRY!

I'm an old man and have known a great many problems, most of which never happened to me.

- Mark Twain

Before developing specific coping strategies, special mention needs to be given to worry. Worry is destructive and wasteful energy. If we can learn to stop worrying, we will gain that energy back to do something about what we were worrying about in the first place.

Convert your useless worrying to **constructive concern**. Being concerned means that you may ask yourself what you can do to improve the situation and then calmly proceed to do it. Being concerned means that you do not engage in self-pity or exhaust your energy mulling over the past. You live in the present and learn to take appropriate action when needed.

Again, the difference between worry and concern is a matter of degree. It is important to be concerned about people and issues. If we let our concerns get out of control to the point of rendering us ineffective, it becomes worrying.

Go to page 84 and complete the Critical Thinking and Application Activity 4–4.

EFFECTIVE COPING STRATEGIES

Remember that the most important aspect of stress is that it is individually determined. Its meaning lies within us. Therefore, we are the ones to determine what is stressful and whether we are going to use stress to our advantage or let it use us. It should logically follow, if *we* determine the level of stress, *we* should be able to control it.

Someone once said that you do not get ulcers from what you eat, but rather from what is eating you. It is important to cope with stress before you suffer from stress overload or burnout. There are two basic ways you can cope with stress. The first is to effectively cope with the emotional side of stress. The second is to deal with its physical side. Stress can wreak havoc on our emotional well-being. However, we can use our minds to control stress and make it a positive influence. The five main strategies to emotionally handle stress include:

- Recognizing and eliminating stressors
- Reframing your thinking
- Using good time management
- Developing a social support group
- Rejuvenating yourself

Recognize and Eliminate Stressors. First, it is important to know what personally stresses *you* out and when you are getting out of control. One simple yet effective method is to write down your stressors. Now think of ways you can regain control over or eliminate the stress completely. However, realize there are some stressors that you can do something about and some that you cannot.

For example, you will eventually be faced with treating a terminally ill patient. A terminal illness is untreatable and irreversible. This certainly causes stress for your patient. The patient may be difficult to deal with, but think of what he or she is going through. This situation can cause stress for you. You cannot change the stress caused by knowing that your patient is going to die. However, you can make a big difference in how your patient dies. Your care and support can increase your patient's quality of life during the remaining time and allow him or her to put personal affairs in order. You can make it the best death possible. Your concern and subsequent actions can truly make a difference.

Reframe Your Thinking. You can also cope with stress by changing how you think about a stressful situation. By **reframing** your perceptions, you can change the meaning of an event. Reframing means to rename in a positive sense. The Chinese word for problem means opportunity. If we can learn to look at what we perceive to be problems as actually opportunities, our stress would reduce drastically.

For example, multiskilling and multicompetencies are two important concepts in health care. This means you may be cross-trained to do other basic jobs. Most allied health professionals are being trained to perform vital sign assessment and basic patient care (e.g., bathing, turning) to assist nursing personnel in units where they may be stationed. As an occupational therapist, this may cause stress because you think it is "not your job" or you are anxious about performing certain skills. However, an excellent occupational therapist would understand the necessity and reframe his or her thinking as follows: This will give me an opportunity to learn new skills that I can add to my résumé. In addition, it will make me more valuable to my organization and increase my job security. Besides, it will be fun to work more hand in hand with the nurses in basic patient care.

Use Good Time Management. You must master the effective time management techniques discussed in Chapter 3 to reduce stress.

Especially, remember to say "no" to additional projects, responsibilities, or demands when accepting them would mean being overcommitted. Note that complaining is not the same as saying no. Complaining does not relieve stress, it reinforces it. By being organized and not allowing your work to pile up, you will greatly reduce the stress in your life.

Develop a Social Support Group. Your family, friends, and teachers can provide support in dealing with stress. Research suggests that emotional support helps people deal with stress. That is why it is so important to develop a social network and spend time with family and friends each week. Even if these are just people you trust to listen to you, this will allow you to vent some of your stress. Their outside objective perceptions may also help the situation. In other words, they may see things you cannot because you are too emotional about the situation.

As a health care practitioner, you become an integral part of the patients' support systems. They rely on your medical expertise to assess and treat their condition. They also rely on your emotional support to help them through their stressful periods.

Rejuvenate Yourself. Learn to rejuvenate or recharge yourself when stress gets the best of you. You can do this in many ways. For example, take a break from your routine and do enjoyable activities or hobbies. Take a mental health vacation (a day or half a day to yourself) or, if you can, a real minivacation. Remember, vacation means to vacate and get away. Do you know people who take vacations and try to cram everything in to a point where they need a vacation after their vacation?

Listening to your favorite music can also help. Research has proven music affects many of the major systems of our body. Music can both stimulate and relax you, depending on the type. It's best to listen to soothing music during periods of excessive stress.

Finally, do not forget to have a good laugh. The average 4-year-old child laughs every few minutes. Laughter helps bring you back in perspective, and besides it feels good. Laughter also helps you physically by lowering blood pressure, releasing endorphins, and stimulating the pleasure centers of the brain. You will notice that patients with a good sense of humor are more compliant and respond better to treatment. Have you ever said to someone, "Someday we'll look back on this and laugh?" Chances are it's funny now, so why wait? Figure 4–5 relates the five effective emotional strategies to deal with stress.

LEARNER:

Go to page 84 and complete the Critical Thinking and Application Activities 4–5, 4–6, and 4–7.

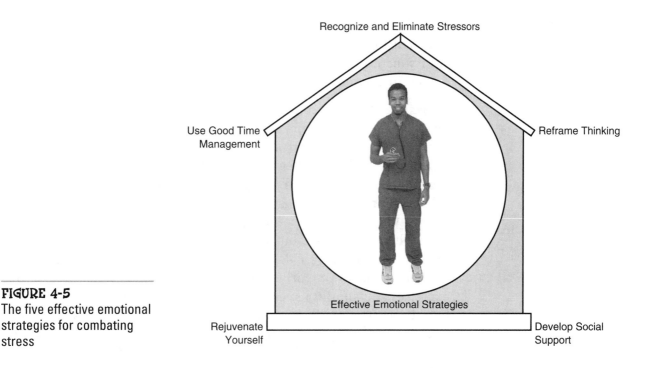

FIGURE 4-5
The five effective emotional strategies for combating stress

EFFECTIVE PHYSICAL STRATEGIES

You cannot separate mind from body. If you mentally feel bad, it affects your physical well-being. If you do not take care of your physical body, you lack energy and focus, cannot sleep, and do not reach your full emotional potential. Therefore, you must balance emotional and physical strategies. Indeed, you will see that some of these techniques help both your physical and emotional health. Handling stress "physically" can be broken down into the following four areas:

- Rest and leisure
- Exercise
- Nutrition
- Relaxation techniques

Rest and Leisure. Adequate sleep is a must for us to function at our peak and handle stress. Research has shown that lack of sleep (sleep deprivation) makes people more susceptible to illness. Of course, lack of sleep also makes people more irritable and less able to focus. Experts recommend that most adults get between 7 to 9 hours of sleep a night.

Taking leisure time for yourself can also help restore your ability to deal with stress. Even if that leisure time is only 15 minutes, it can help greatly. Sometimes, the more you focus on a major problem, the more stress it causes. This is a good time to take a break and get away from the problem by doing something else. In many cases, the solution will then just come to you as if by magic. It is not magic, just your subconscious mind working for you. This phenomenon is discussed in Chapter 5.

Exercise. Physical exercise and sports are a great way to work off tensions of everyday life. It helps you gain both a physical and mental focus if done properly. Any type of aerobic activity exercises your muscles and relieves mental tension. Vigorous walking, jogging, running, bicycling, and lifting weights are all things you can do by yourself. Of course, you can also find a good workout partner or play team sports. Vigorous exercise also releases a group of hormones called endorphins. These are our body's natural painkillers. They also are mood-elevating chemicals that give us a healthy natural high.

Remember to properly warm up and stretch before any vigorous exercise. You should never stretch "cold" muscles (i.e., muscles that have been inactive). You can march in place, step side to side, or take a walk to warm up your muscles. After the warm-up, you should do your stretches. Stretching not only helps prevent injuries but also helps relieve muscular tension and lower blood pressure. Follow certain rules when stretching. First, never rush through the stretches by bouncing or using fast, jerky movements that could strain or tear muscles. Stretch slowly until you feel mild tension and then hold the position for 10 to 30 seconds.

Nutrition. Good nutrition is a must for our growth and development. It also aids us in fighting stress and disease. In addition, it is a good idea to drink plenty of water. Water makes up most of our body. Water aids in digestion, absorption of nutrients, and removal of waste products. Even though water is found in most foods, you should drink 6 to 8 glasses every day for good health.

Cut down on caffeine, which is found in coffee, tea, and many sodas. Caffeine is a potent central nervous system stimulant. Large amounts can make you anxious, nervous, and unable to get a good night's sleep.

Certain foods have been found to have a calming effect on the body. Foods high in complex carbohydrates (whole grains, beans, seeds, nuts, fruits, and vegetables) have been shown to increase levels of serotonin. Serotonin is a chemical in the brain that helps you feel more relaxed.

Relaxation Techniques. Practicing relaxation techniques will help clear your mind and make you sharper. Most people will find a million excuses why they cannot take the time to relax. Do you see the illogical thinking? If they are *that busy,* then they need to take the time to relax and restore their body and mind. This time also allows you to listen to your body. Two types of relaxation techniques that are effective are breathing relaxation and meditation techniques.

Slow and deep breathing serves several purposes. First, it increases oxygen to your brain and body. It also slows down your thinking to help clear your head and relax your muscles.

Specific techniques are given at the end of this chapter.

What Do YOU Think?

Breathing and Stress Reduction

Breathing is something we do automatically, with little or no thought. An individual takes about 20,000 breaths every 24 hours. We are learning that the more we pay attention to our breathing, the better it can help reduce stress. The medical profession and many athletic programs are incorporating ancient yoga breathing techniques in their treatment or training programs.

Yoga breathing is fast becoming a part of mainstream medical practices and is used in stress reduction workshops. Pranayama (pra-nah-YAH-mah), a system of ancient breathing techniques that slows the heart, lowers blood pressure, and relieves stress, has been proven effective.

Yoga breathing teaches you to relax the diaphragm, the main muscle of breathing. Some cardiac rehabilitation programs teach this technique to reduce the stress on the heart and increase oxygen intake from the lungs. In addition, patients with chronic obstructive pulmonary disease (COPD) have been taught this technique to treat their shortness of breath and anxiety when the disease flares up.

Meditation techniques can vary greatly. Meditation is basically focusing your attention while clearing your mind of all its constant chattering. You can also use visual or guided imagery to replace troubling thoughts and constant mind chatter with relaxing thoughts and pleasant images. One other related technique is progressive muscle relaxation.

You will get a chance to practice these techniques in the critical thinking and applications activities at the end of this chapter. Give each a try. You may find some work better for you than others. Practice and use whatever works best for you. These techniques take only 10 to 15 minutes per day, yet they can make your day much more productive. Table 4–2 contrasts some of the do's and don'ts of stress management.

TABLE 4-2
Do's and Don'ts of Stress Management

DO	DON'T
Confront a problem	Think it will resolve itself
Discuss things calmly	Fight or yell
Exercise	Lie around, bite nails
Accept responsibility	Blame others
Use relaxation techniques	Use alcohol or drugs
Accept/learn from your mistakes	Be a perfectionist
Keep good nutrition	Overeat or undereat
Be concerned	Worry
Live in the present	Agonize over the past or future
Help others	Avoid people

SUMMARY

Stress is a factor in all our lives. The health care profession can be especially stressful. However, *good stress* can help us perform better, whereas *bad stress* can have a negative impact on our performance. Continual high levels of stress can lead to several health problems. This chapter discusses three steps in order to use stress as a motivator and an enhancer. The first step is to assess and recognize your personal stress signals and stress producers. Then, you can develop specific coping strategies that will work for you. A third important step is to differentiate the state of worry from being concerned about a situation.

LEARNER:

Go to page 85 and complete the Critical Thinking and Application Activities 4–8, 4–9, 4–10, and 4–11.

Why These Activities Are Important to You

Stress is something we must all learn to deal with. Many people do not realize that stress can be used as a positive force if managed correctly. These activities will help you learn how to cope with and harness your stress in a positive way. The health care environment will certainly give you much practice in dealing with stress. Besides, if you can't handle stress, what kind of message does that send to your patient?

Types of Stress

This chapter discusses the different types of stress. Most notably, you can have good stress that gets you "up" and makes you sharp for the task at hand. You can also have bad stress that inhibits your ability to do well.

The key point is how you perceive the stress and whether you control it, or it controls you. Let us begin by exploring the types of stress in your life.

CRITICAL THINKING AND APPLICATION ACTIVITIES

4-1 Questions about Stress

1. Identify three situations where stress was a positive experience for you.

   a. _____

   b. _____

   c. _____

2. Why do people who think negatively experience a lot of stress?

   _____

   _____

3. How do you know when you are getting stressed out?

   _____

   _____

4. List five physical signs you have when experiencing negative stress.

   a. _____

   b. _____

   c. _____

   d. _____

   e. _____

4-2 Sources of Stress

This chapter describes a three-point system for stress management. We will now work on the first point, which is recognizing your stress signals and producers.

Your stress signals are your early warning detection system that says you have to do something. That something will come soon. For now, learn to identify the sources of stress in your life and recognize the signals when stress is out of control.

Stress can come from several different sources. For example, it can come from your personal life, work, or school. Identify two major sources that produce stress in your personal life and two sources of stress in school.

1. Personal stressor 1: _____

2. Personal stressor 2: _____

3. School stressor 1: _____

4. School stressor 2: _____

Your Physical Signs of Stress

For each personal and school stressor list three physical symptoms you experience when the stress gets excessive.

1. Personal stressor 1: _____

2. Personal stressor 2: _____

3. School stressor 1: _____

4. School stressor 2: _____

Turning Worry into Concern

Now we move on to the second point of the three-point system. Avoid worry! Although a very short section was devoted to "worrying" in this chapter, it is one of the most destructive activities we can engage in. Worrying does nothing but wear us down both physically and mentally. However, being concerned means that we calmly analyze the situation and do what is needed to be done to improve it.

1. Write down the one thing you worry the most about. Be specific. Remember, worry is when "it kind of drives you crazy thinking about it."

   _____

2. Now write down what you can do about it. In other words, what steps can be taken to improve the situation? Again, be specific.

   _____

3. Now write down what *you are* going to do about it. Your answer should be pretty much the same as that for the previous question. Do you get the point I am emphasizing?

   _____

4. Finally, write down when you are going to start doing it! _____

   Notice there is not much room for your response. This emphasizes the point to *do* something about your worrying and to do it *now*. Appropriate and timely action will make your life a lot more fun and productive. It will also slow down that constant mind talk we all do, which speeds up a zillion times when we worry.

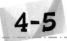

Reframing Your Thinking

The third and final point is to develop effective emotional and physical coping strategies to use when stress gets out of hand. Some may work better for you than others. However, you must develop some on both the physical and emotional sides for balance. This section deals with emotional coping mechanisms.

How you perceive a situation makes all the difference in the world. For each of the following negative perceptions, rewrite in a positive frame of mind.

Example:

Negative: *I failed this test, I will never do well in this class!*

Positive: *I failed this test, but I can do better next time and pull my grade up. I will learn from my mistakes and improve my study skills and get a good grade on the next test.*

Negative: *I cannot get along well with others. I'll never have any really good friends.*

Positive: _____

Negative: *I do not have any free time to myself. I'll never get everything done and have time for me.*

Positive: _____

_____

Negative: *I do not like the way I look.*

Positive: _____

_____

Developing a Social Support Group

Draw a positive picture of yourself, or paste a good photo in the center of the page. Now draw several ovals around the picture and write in the names of your social support group. Include teachers, family members, and friends. Your support group may also include members of your community.

How Do You Recharge Yourself?

1. List five things you like to do that take your mind off of stress and makes you feel good. Substance abuse does *not* count because we all know that over time, it destroys us and those around us. Remember, the things you choose can do no harm to yourself or others.

   _____ Read
   _____ Write
   _____ Watch TV or Movie
   _____ Play Xbox
   _____ Cuddle with my doggies ☺

2. How many times did you do each activity last week? Place this number next to each activity. Could you have done it more? Can you think of all the excuses why you did not? Remember to take care of yourself and enjoy life.

How Do You Do with Exercise and Nutrition?

Answer the following questions and come up with a plan to improve any *no* responses.

Example:

Do you exercise three times a week for at least 30 minutes each session? *No*

Plan: *I will develop a schedule that will have three sessions of exercise per week. Because I like to ride my bike, one session will be bicycling for 30–40 min. This will also help clear my mind.*

1. Do you drink 6 to 8 glasses of drinking water per day?

   Plan: _____

   _____

2. Do you follow a good nutritional program?

   Plan: _____

   _____

3. Do you eat in moderation?

    Plan: _____

    _____

4. Do you limit your caffeine intake?

    Plan: _____

    _____

5. Do you avoid substance abuse such as nicotine, alcohol, or illegal street drugs?

    Plan: _____

    _____

 ## Relaxation Techniques

These final activities deal with physical coping mechanisms of stress. This section focuses on some re-laxation techniques that will help both your physical and emotional well-being. Try them all and see which ones work best for you. Then devote at least 15 minutes a day using one or more technique. The ideal system is two 15-minute sessions, one in the morning and one before bed.

Practice the following techniques daily for 1 week. Then describe how they make you feel afterwards. Keep doing the ones that work best for you.

Technique 1: Breathing Relaxation

1. Lie on a comfortable floor on your back with palms up. Make sure there are no distractions.
2. Now inhale slowly through your nostrils as deeply as you can for 3 to 4 seconds. Fill your lungs, drawing the air in as your abdomen rises. Focus on your abdomen rising and your breathing, and think of nothing else.
3. Hold your breath for 3 to 4 seconds.
4. Then, with your lips slightly open, exhale through your mouth slowly. Breathe normally a few times, and then take another deep breath. Take 10 deep breaths in all.

Describe how you feel: _____

Technique 2: Visual Imagery

Visual imagery is a technique that allows you to actually picture yourself "relaxed." Visualization or guided imagery is a form of daydreaming.

1. Get in a comfortable position. This can be lying down or in a recliner chair.
2. Close your eyes and take a few deep breaths to calm yourself.
3. Form a clear image in your mind of a pleasant scene, such as a mountaintop, waterfall, or any other place you find relaxing. The idea is to try to engage as many of your senses as possible, imagining the smells, sounds, tastes, and feelings in the scene.

Describe how you feel: _____

NOTE: A variation of this is to use technique one, and as you exhale, visually imagine all the stress flowing from your body.

Technique 3: Meditation

Meditation simply means focusing your attention.

1. Again sit or lie in a comfortable position.
2. Take a slow deep breath (with stomach) and repeat, either aloud or silently, a syllable, a word, or a small group of words that have a positive meaning.

NOTE: A variation is to gaze at a fixed object, such as a candle, and focus all your thoughts on this object. The key is to not think about anything or to let your mind start talking to you. You can meditate in as little as 5 minutes, although 15 to 20 minutes is optimal for relaxation.

Describe how you feel: _____

Technique 4: Progressive Relaxation

Progressive muscle relaxation is where you alternately tighten and then relax your muscles. It is a great way to release tension and may even help treat tension headaches.

1. Alternately tense (hold to count of five) and then relax the major muscle groups in your body.

2. Start with your feet, then legs, thighs, buttocks, abdomen, and so on, up to your head.

3. When you release the tension in each group, silently say to yourself, "relax and let go," or use visual imagery to imagine the tension flowing from those muscles.

Describe how you feel: _____

4-10 Case Study

David has an average of two severe headaches per week. Having read about stress management, he began to become more aware of his reaction to stress in his life. He noticed that when he began to get "worked up" he would chew on his pencil and a little later his neck muscles would tighten. After a while, his stomach would then get upset, and eventually he would end up with a headache. Do you have any suggestions for David? Do you think he could reduce the number of headaches he experiences? Explain a positive action plan for David that emphasizes early intervention.

_____
_____
_____
_____

4-11 Internet Activities

Using Internet search engines, find additional material on stress management that can help you and your fellow students. Some suggested keywords are: stress management, harmful effects of stress, depression, worry, meditation, and nutrition. Write down something new that you found to share.

_____
_____
_____
_____

THOUGHTS TO PONDER

Don't cry over spilt milk.

- ???

A ship in port is safe, but that is not what ships are built for.

- ???

It is not easy to find happiness in ourselves, and it is not possible to find it elsewhere.

- Agnes Repplier, from the Treasure Chest

Most folks are about as happy as they make up their minds to be.

- Abraham Lincoln

CHAPTER 5

Thinking and Reasoning Skills

OBJECTIVES

Upon completion of this chapter, you should be able to:

Define and differentiate the different types of thinking.

Begin to integrate critical and creative thinking skills into *your* life.

Use an effective decision-making process to maximize your chances for success.

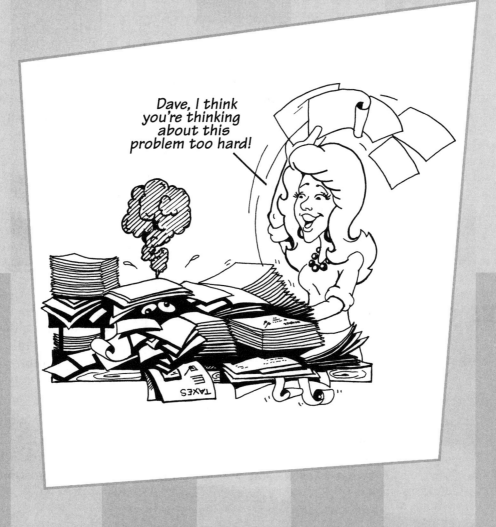

Dave, I think you're thinking about this problem too hard!

KEY TERMS

analogy
brainstorming
cognitive processes
creative thinking
critical thinking

decision making
deductive reasoning
directed thinking
inductive reasoning
lateral thinking

logical thinking
undirected thinking
vertical thinking

INTRODUCTION

> **W**hether you think you can or think you can't—
> you're probably right.
>
> - Henry Ford

Have you ever "thought" about how you "think"? Psychologists, who specialize in studying how humans think, use the term **cognitive processes** to refer to the complex mental activities that compose thinking. These mental activities include using language, reasoning, solving problems, conceptualizing, remembering, imagining, and learning verbal material. These cognitive processes help us respond to our environment and greatly influence how we behave.

Several different types of "thinking" have been classified. These may include **logical**, **critical**, **creative**, **directed**, and **undirected thinking**. We discuss these thinking types individually and then relate how they can be integrated to make you an effective thinker. As an effective thinker, you will be able to maximize your decision-making and problem-solving skills. The development of these thinking skills will in turn make you an excellent health care practitioner.

TYPES OF THINKING

We use logic several times each day. Any time we evaluate, judge, or decide something, we must rely on our logical thinking. Just what is logic? It is your ability to reason in a given situation. If you are cold, you will figure out a way to become warm. Your logic may tell you to get a coat, go inside, build a fire, or turn up the thermostat. You will choose what you think is the best response given the situation and your previous knowledge. For example, if you did not know what a thermostat was, it could not be one of your options. So one part of logic relies on your past experience and knowledge. Another part of logical thinking relies on your ability to reason deductively and inductively.

Deductive reasoning is a form of logical thinking in which you reach a true conclusion based on true facts called premises. For example, you may have the following premises:

Premise: Patients with advanced lung disease will experience shortness of breath (SOB) on exertion.

Premise: Bob has advanced lung disease and is trying to help his daughter move.

Conclusion: Bob will experience SOB while helping his daughter move.

In this example, you used deductive reasoning to reach a true conclusion. The conclusion in deductive reasoning is always true if the premises are true. Because of your use of deductive reasoning, you can assist Bob by teaching him breathing retraining exercises and teaching him how and when to use his supplemental oxygen to breathe more effectively. This will decrease his SOB and make the moving day go a whole lot better.

In the previous example, you have just taken action that could prevent a potential crisis such as a cardiac arrest for Bob. This is called proactive thinking, or thinking ahead so that you are not in a crisis situation. Many people wait for the problem to occur and then react to the crisis. This is called reactive thinking. Which do you think is better?

Another type of logical thinking is **inductive reasoning**. Here you make your best guess based on the premises or facts. Your conclusion has a high probability of being true but is not always true. Here is an example of inductive reasoning:

Premise: People who smoke have an increased risk of getting lung cancer.

Premise: Mary smoked two packs of cigarettes for 20 years.

Conclusion: Mary will get lung cancer.

Although Mary's risk of getting lung cancer is much greater than that of someone who has not smoked and although it is possible that Mary may get lung cancer, the conclusion may not be true. She may never develop lung cancer. She may die from emphysema first or there may be several other possible outcomes. However, if she enters the emergency department with signs and symptoms that are consistent with cancer, your inductive reasoning, coupled with her past medical history, would lead you to suspect and test for the occurrence of lung cancer.

LEARNER:

Go to page 103 and complete the Critical Thinking and Application Activities 5–1 and 5–2.

CRITICAL AND CREATIVE THINKING

Much attention is being paid to developing critical thinking skills in students. However, there are many definitions and views on critical thinking, making this concept confusing. One definition of critical thinking is "the ability to suspend judgment, to consider alternatives, to analyze and evaluate." Another definition states "purposeful, goal-directed thinking," and there are still several other definitions. However, these definitions all include several thinking skills such as the ability to develop a hypothesis, to test and rate possible solutions, and to maintain an objective viewpoint. Critical thinking skills relate to analytical thinking—the ability to objectively analyze a situation or set of facts. It should be noted that critical thinking skills (like all thinking skills) can be developed and improved on through practice.

Creative thinking also has several definitions and many misconceptions surrounding it. One common misconception is that creativity is only for artists, musicians, and writers. If we simply define creative thinking as "the generation of ideas that results in the improvement of the efficiency or the effectiveness of the system," we can see that it relates to all of us. Psychologists who devote themselves to the study of the mind define creativity as the ability to see things in a new way and to help in problem solving. A worker who develops a better way to do the job, a parent who helps his or her child to learn a new skill or overcome a problem, and even someone who finds a better route on a map are all being creative. We use this skill every day of our lives without being fully aware of it.

Edward De Bono, an expert on thinking, coined the terms **vertical thinking** and **lateral thinking** to contrast critical and creative thinking. Vertical thinking relies on logic and each idea relates to the next. Vertical thinking allows us to make assumptions based on past experiences and relies on logical thinking, which includes deductive and inductive reasoning, which we have already discussed. Remember how we went in a stepwise fashion from premise to premise to conclusion?

Lateral thinking creates new ideas by making connections with no set pathway. Lateral thinking takes stored information and relates it in a previously unrelated manner. It generates the ideas that will later be evaluated by vertical, or logical, thinking modes. Some people think of this as "sideways thinking" because you are making connections with other thoughts versus the vertical step-by-step thinking. Figure 5–1 (appears on page 93) contrasts vertical and lateral thinking.

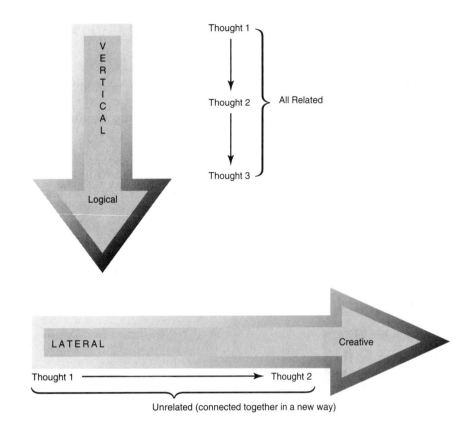

FIGURE 5-1
Contrasting vertical and lateral thinking

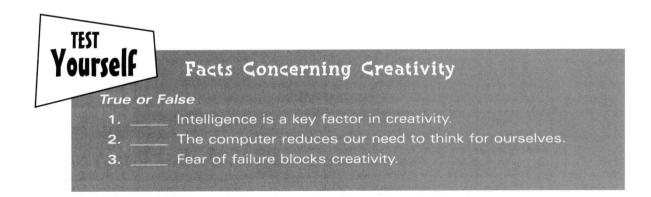

What Do YOU Think?

Integrating Critical and Creative Thinking

Although these thinking styles are usually discussed separately, to be a truly effective thinker you must learn to use both. Working in health care demands that you can use your critical thinking skills to analyze a patient or situation and then use your creative thinking skills to come up with a possible solution or treatments. You must then return to your critical thinking skills to evaluate the outcomes. Look at this quote and decide what you think it is saying.

The diversity and complexity of nursing practice in today's healthcare field make it necessary to prepare nurses who can think critically and creatively and who have a sound education in nursing science, related sciences and the Humanities. (From a report presented to the American Association of Colleges of Nursing.)

Can you see the importance of developing both critical and creative thinking skills?

TEST Yourself

Facts Concerning Creativity

True or False

1. _____ Intelligence is a key factor in creativity.
2. _____ The computer reduces our need to think for ourselves.
3. _____ Fear of failure blocks creativity.

DIRECTED AND UNDIRECTED THINKING

Most thinking is hard to categorize, and with all the terms, it can get quite confusing. One classification system simplifies thinking in terms of contrasting directed and undirected thinking. Both directed and undirected thinking involve some of the same mental processes such as memory, imagination, and association. Directed thinking is usually highly controllable, and a conscious effort is made to solve a specific problem or situation. The processes of learning, reasoning, and decision making are good examples of directed thinking.

Undirected thinking is more loose and free flowing. Dreaming can be thought of as a type of undirected thinking process. This can include both daydreaming and dreaming while asleep. There is no apparent goal or specific problem, just a steady stream of thought. However, you will soon learn that this type of thinking can also assist in problem solving.

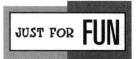

JUST FOR FUN

Brain Teasers

1. If an electric train was traveling northwest on a railroad track in Greenland, in which direction would the smoke blow? <u>Electric train doesn't blow smoke.</u>

2. I have two coins and one is not a nickel. They total 55 cents. What are the two coins? <u>The other one is a nickel</u>

3. Count the number of squares in Figure 5–2. <u>30</u>

FIGURE 5-2
How many squares?

LEARNER:

Go to page 104 and complete the Critical Thinking and Application Activities 5–3 and 5–4.

THE TOTAL THINKING PROCESS

DECISIONS

Decisions are something we make every day of our lives. Just what is **decision making**? Decision making is the act of making an informed choice between a number of alternatives to solve a problem or maximize an opportunity. Decision making helps you develop a definite course of action. Just look at some of the decisions you will make in a day.

We have to decide what time to get up, what clothes to wear, what we are going to do that day, what to eat, and so on. Many decisions have short-term effects and do not require a specific process. For example, you do not have to go through several steps in the decision-making process to decide what to eat. Usually, you look at the menu, decide what you like and how much you can spend, and then place your order. This is a short-term decision that will not have long-term effects, except maybe some nausea if the food was not prepared properly.

However, decisions that have long-term effects on our lives should have a specific process to maximize their successful outcome. For example, the following questions will all greatly influence your future:

What are my studying strategies?

What courses should I take to prepare for my career?

How do I maintain a healthy lifestyle?

Using the decision-making process will help you make more informed decisions that will lead to the results you desire. Decision making also helps *you* control the direction of your life instead of letting events or others take control of you. Decision making has some risks involved, however; it makes you confront your problems and take action that will minimize any risks.

THE DECISION-MAKING PROCESS

The decision-making process can be called many things. Some refer to it as problem solving, but this makes it seem as if everything is a problem to be solved, which is not always the case. Sometimes you are looking at maximizing an opportunity, choosing the right path, creating a new opportunity, and yes, solving a problem. There are several variations of the decision-making process or problem solving, as some may call it, but they all have basically the same five steps:

1. Define the opportunity for positive change.
2. Generate ideas concerning the opportunity.
3. Evaluate your ideas and select the best one.
4. Implement your chosen strategy.
5. Evaluate the impact and modify accordingly.

Now you will examine each of these steps individually and in greater depth. Figure 5–3 shows the steps in the decision-making process.

Step One: Define the Opportunity. Step one is to define the opportunity for positive change. Note that the first step does *not* say define the problem. This is because how you present this first step to your mind will greatly influence the outcome. So by looking at each major decision or problem as an opportunity for positive change, you are already on your way to a great solution.

Using this approach for the first step also increases proactive versus reactive thinking. Reactive thinking is when you wait for a problem to exist and then "react" and try to solve it. This is not very effective because now you may be dealing with a crisis situation that may be difficult to resolve. Proactive thinking is "looking ahead" and preventing problems from occurring. Now you can assess and optimize your environment with calm thinking and prevent many crisis situations from occurring.

You should be able to clearly state what the opportunity is in a manner that shows a positive outcome. Remember, how we state the problem *greatly* influences the rest of the process!

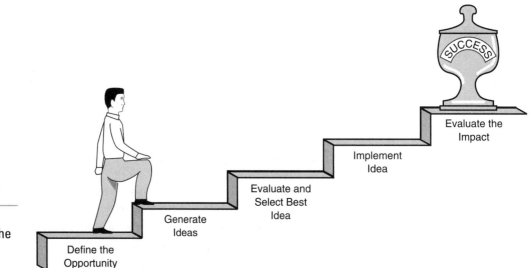

FIGURE 5-3
The five steps in the decision-making process

Here is a common "problem" stated in the sometimes hectic world of health care: "I'm too busy."

The opportunity is not clearly stated, nor does it show any positive outcome. A problem stated in this manner is unlikely to be solved, and the person will only become more frustrated in time and always perceive themselves as too busy and take no action to solve this. However, this can be restated as follows: "How do we streamline work habits to get the work done on time and allow professional development?"

Notice how this now presents an opportunity for professional development to occur when solutions are implemented to get the work done by streamlining work habits. You may find that there are several legitimate shortcuts that can be taken and not compromise high-quality care. This statement will force you to look at the way things are done and try to find better ways to do them. The reward will not be more work piled on, but rather time freed up for professional development, which is crucial in the health care professions.

Here is one more example of a complaint from nonphysician health care members: "Physicians never listen to us."

Look how poorly this problem is stated. First, it implies that they are "never" listened to, which cannot be accurate. Second, using the term *never* leads you to believe that no solution exists. Do you suspect that the person who says this may not have a very positive attitude, which may be part of the problem? A better restatement would be as follows: "How do we develop strategies to increase positive physician communication and interaction?"

This now clearly states what is hoped will be accomplished and what the positive outcomes will be.

After having clearly stated the opportunity, you now need to gather all the pertinent data before going on to the next step, which will generate possible solutions. Get all the facts you can that relate to this opportunity. For example, if you were a supervisor and had a problem employee, your "opportunity" would be to achieve a positive change and have a happy productive employee. You would have to gather all the facts available as to why this employee is being unproductive before coming up with ideas. In summation, clearly state the opportunity with a positive outcome and gather all the "facts" together in step one. This step may take some time, but it will lay a solid foundation for success in your decision-making process.

LEARNER:

Go to page 105 and complete the Critical Thinking and Application Activities 5–5 and 5–6.

Step Two: Generate Ideas. Step two is to generate ideas concerning the opportunity. Now is the time to use your creative thinking skills and come up with ideas concerning the opportunity. It is important not to judge any of these ideas as good or bad. The key to this step is coming up with a quantity of ideas. Even what may seem to be far out ideas should be encouraged at this step.

How good are you at generating new ideas? If you consider yourself poor at this, you are not alone. Many people feel they are uncreative, but nothing could be farther from the truth. We are all creative, and there are ways we can enhance this creativity.

A lot of research was done concerning the left and right sides of our brain and creativity. It has been shown that the left side of our brain is more analytical, whereas the right side is more intuitive and creative. Some people have contended that creative individuals think mainly with the right side of the brain, whereas more logical or analytical thinkers are controlled by the left side of the brain. This was shown to be an oversimplification of what was actually occurring. During positron emission testing (which can measure and locate brain activity) of individuals performing creative tasks, the brain's electrical activity flickered between both hemispheres. This demonstrated the need, even in creative tasks, of connecting the right and left brain hemispheres. Therefore, it is important to make these cross-connections to enhance creative thinking. There are several techniques to enhance this.

ASSOCIATIVE THINKING AND VISUALIZATION. One method to force "cross-connections" is to sketch your opportunity or issue in the center of your paper. This is referred to as developing a concept map. Next, print key words and ideas and connect these to your central issue. Use colors and symbols to emphasize certain points. Study this visual picture and see if you can find new relationships, patterns, or ideas. It may take time, but the more ideas you develop, the better chance for a successful solution. Figure 5–4 is a visualization of a successful health career.

BRAINSTORMING. **Brainstorming** is a powerful way to enhance creativity. This is when a small group of people (five to eight) collaborate and come up with ideas concerning an opportunity or issue that has been presented to them. However, it can be done with only two or more people. If done properly, it uses several brains that have different experiences, knowledge, and insights to greatly enhance the creative power. There are three important rules to make sure this process is effective.

RULE NUMBER ONE: WITHHOLD PREMATURE CRITICISMS. Have you ever had someone be critical of an idea you gave in front of a group by saying something or using body language such as eye rolling? How did it make you feel? Did you want to give another idea?

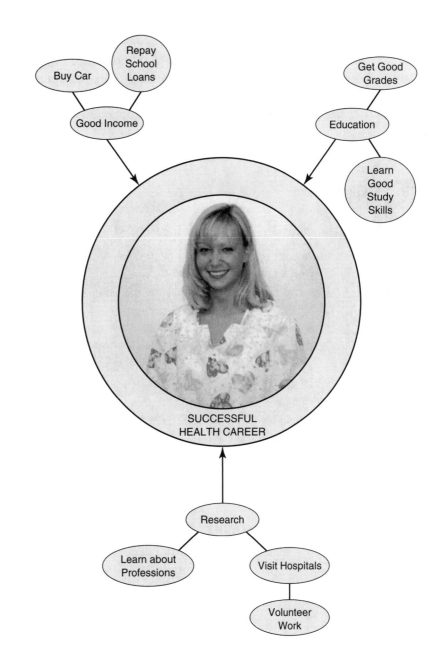

FIGURE 5-4
Associative thinking and
visualization

Premature criticism will kill the creative process and should be avoided at all costs. Any idea, no matter how far-fetched, should be considered. Remember, the goal is not to come up with the best solution at this time. The goal here is to list all kinds of ideas that will be analyzed and evaluated in the next step. You might even combine some ideas at this stage.

RULE NUMBER TWO: THE QUANTITY OF IDEAS IS IMPORTANT AT THIS STAGE, NOT THE QUALITY. The more ideas generated, the better the odds that a high-quality idea will emerge. Sometimes we are conditioned to believe that there is only one right answer and not being "right" means failure. This may be true in math, but in creative thinking, there are no "right" or "wrong" answers, only ideas.

RULE NUMBER THREE: GET RID OF DISTRACTIONS. A nonthreatening atmosphere that is free of distractions provides the best environment for creative thinking. Distractions include noise, poor lighting, squeaky chairs, a telephone, pager, or a room that is either too hot or too cold.

What Do YOU Think?

Barriers to the Creative Process

Listed below are some barriers to the creative process. Think about which ones may apply to you. Checkmark the ones you need to work on.

1. _____ Fear of losing control: Are you threatened by allowing others to give ideas because you feel you may not be "in charge"?

2. _____ Resistance to change: When change is proposed, do you feel "this is the way it always has been done, why should we look for a better way?"

3. _____ Premature criticism: Do you immediately judge someone else's idea as good or bad?

4. _____ "Borrowing of ideas": Do you take credit for others' ideas? Do you think people would give additional ideas to a person who they think will take the credit?

5. _____ Procedural dependency: Do you think that there must be only one right way to do something?

ANALOGIES. An **analogy** forces cross-connections between two unlike things. This can be helpful in generating ideas that would not have been thought of otherwise. Coors was paying millions of dollars to dispose of beer by-products, and creative consultants were brought in to come up with ideas. They used the analogy of Tom Sawyer, who convinced his friends that painting a fence was a privilege they should pay for. Coors employees used this analogy to come up with the idea to sell their beer by-products to the Japanese cattle industry. They now took something that was costly to dispose of and actually turned it into a profit much as Tom Sawyer convinced his friends it was a privilege to do his chore.

Many inventions came about as a result of analogies. Velcro was discovered because an inventor got a bunch of sticky burrs on his pants while walking through the woods. Analyzing the burrs, he developed Velcro, which has hundreds of uses. Using analogies can be both fun and creative in developing unique solutions.

LEARNER:

Go to page 106 and complete the Critical Thinking and Application Activities 5–7, 5–8, 5–9, 5–10, and 5–11.

Step Three: Evaluate and Select Best Idea. Step three is to evaluate your ideas and select the best one. In this step, you shift to your logical or analytical thinking to evaluate each idea or combination of ideas for its successful outcomes. Basically, you are weighing the pros and cons of each idea in order to choose the best idea that will give you your desired outcome.

You now need to select or choose from among the various ideas, the course of action that will provide the greatest chance for success. You can visually test each of them by imagining that each has already been put into effect. Consider the short- and long-term effects of each idea. Evaluate their merit and then make your choice.

LEARNER:

Go to page 108 and complete the Critical Thinking and Application Activity 5–12.

Step Four: Implement the Idea. Step four is to implement your chosen strategy. This is when you put your idea into action. Here, you must ask several questions: What is the best way to implement your chosen solution? What factors may have to be considered in this implementation process? How do you need to communicate this idea and to whom? Once it is implemented, you can proceed to Step five.

Step Five: Evaluate Impact. Step five is to evaluate the impact of your idea and modify it accordingly. Does your chosen idea create the positive opportunity or solve the problem? Is the outcome desirable? If the solution is not desirable, consider another one, rethink all possible solutions, or reevaluate the problem. Get feedback from as many sources as possible to determine whether your idea is having a positive impact. The more feedback you receive, the better your ability to evaluate and modify the outcomes.

The five steps to the decision-making process may seem like a lot to go through, but it is well worth the effort. With practice, these steps will become second nature and will be used almost effortlessly. Besides, you are worth the best effort when making the truly important decisions, which will have a major impact on your life.

SUMMARY

Thinking is something you do every day of your life. Understanding the various types of thinking will make you better able to analyze a situation and develop an effective idea or solution. The decision-making process combines the various types of thinking into an effective strategy for problem solving. The five steps to the decision-making process are:

1. Define the opportunity for positive change.
2. Generate ideas concerning the opportunity.

3. Evaluate your ideas and select the best one.

4. Implement your chosen strategy.

5. Evaluate the impact and modify your idea accordingly.

Learning about and practicing these steps will make you an excellent decision maker.

LEARNER:

Go to page 110 and complete the Critical Thinking and Application Activities 5–13, 5–14, and 5–15.

Why These Activities Are Important to You

Thinking is something we do every day. Good thinking skills are critical for a future health care practitioner. You must be able to assess, diagnose, develop, and implement treatment plans. In addition, decision-making and problem-solving skills must be sharply honed to effectively deal with situations that can arise daily. We can all become better thinkers with practice.

CRITICAL THINKING AND APPLICATION ACTIVITIES

5-1 Logical Thinking

1. Define logical thinking in your own terms.

   _____

   _____

2. List three people you know personally whom you consider to be logical.

   _____

   _____

   _____

3. What is it about these individuals that led you to call them logical? List some personal attributes that you feel contribute to their logical thought process. Write a short paragraph for each individual to answer this question.

   _____

   _____

   _____

   _____

   _____

   _____

   _____

4. Interview at least one of these individuals and list five reasons why that person believes that he or she is a "logical person."

   a. _____

   b. _____

   c. _____

   d. _____

   e. _____

5-2 Deductive and Inductive Thinking

1. Write your definition of deductive thinking.

   _____

   _____

2. Give an example of two premises and a deductive conclusion that you have used in your life.

   Premise 1: _____

   Premise 2: _____

   Conclusion: _____

3. Write your definition of inductive thinking.

_____

_____

4. Give an example of two premises and an inductive conclusion that you have used in your life.

Premise 1: _____

Premise 2: _____

Conclusion: _____

5. Research three premises that would support this conclusion: Smoking has been scientifically shown to be detrimental to your health. Is this an inductive or deductive conclusion?

Premise 1: _____

Premise 2: _____

Conclusion: _____

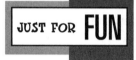 Use your deductive thinking skills to solve this problem:

A cat, a small dog, a goat, and a horse are named Angel, Beauty, King, and Rover. Using the clues that follow, find each animal's name.

Clue 1: King is smaller than both the dog and Rover.

Clue 2: The horse is younger than Angel and Beauty.

Clue 3: Beauty is the oldest and is a good friend of the dog.

Cat's name: _King_   Goat's name: _Beauty_

Dog's name: _Angel_   Horse's name: _Rover_

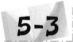 **Contrasting Critical and Creative Thinking**

In today's information age, everyone has access to a vast amount of knowledge. However, the successful people will be able not only to access this information, but also to use their critical and creative thinking skills to develop breakthrough ideas and solutions. Research shows that critical and creative thinking skills can be taught and are key factors in personal and organizational excellence.

1. Define critical and creative thinking in your own words.

Critical thinking: _____

Creative thinking: _____

2. State whether you think the words listed below best reflect critical or creative thinking, or both.

Imagination: _____   Obtaining a medical history: _____

Analytical: _____   Evaluation: _____

Generative: _____   Problem solving: _____

Selective: _____   Brainstorming: _____

Assessment: _____   Daydreaming: _____

Diagnosis: _____

3. Circle any of the preceding words that are examples of directed thinking, and place a star by any examples of undirected thinking.

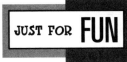

This is an interesting test of your mental flexibility and creativity. Many people report that the answers come to them after they put the test aside. This concept is discussed in the section on creative thinking in problem solving. For now, just have fun and see how many answers you can get.

Instructions: Each equation contains initials of words that will make it correct. For example, "7 = N. of D. in a W." would be 7 = *number* of *days* in a *week*. Now try the rest.

26 = L. of the A.: _26 = letters of alphabet_

12 = S. of the Z.: _12 = signs of the zodiac_

52 = C. in a D. (without the Js): _52 = cards in a deck_

9 = P. in the S. S.: _9 = Plants in the solar system_

88 = P. K.: _88 = Piano keys_

18 = H. on a G. C.: _18 = holes in a golf cours_

29 = D. in F. in a L. Y.: _29 = days in Fed in a Leap year_

1 = W. on a U.: _1 = wheels on a unicycle_

3 = B. M. (S. H. T. R.): _3 = Blind Mice (see how they run)_

4 = Q. in a G.: _4 = quarts in a gallon_

8 = S. on a S. S.: _8 = Sides on a stop sign_

See if you can come up with five on your own to share with your classmates.

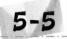 ## Creative Assessment

List five things that you consider to be creative achievements in your life.

a. _Decorating my appartment_

b. _Starting & finishing 5 kids 20+ page scrapbooks_

c. _Shooting both my brother & sisters senior photos_

d. _being a good doggie mom when it came to big med decisions_

e. _____

5-5 Step One: Defining Your Opportunity for Positive Change

Pick one professional opportunity and one personal opportunity and state each in a positive manner. For example, the professional opportunity could be as follows: "How can I prepare myself to succeed in my chosen health career?" Notice that the opportunity is defined and stated in a positive manner. Even a personal problem can be stated in positive manner. For example, "How can I resolve the conflict with my coworker so that our work hours can be more enjoyable and productive?" Notice the positive opportunity? This is a lot better than, "Why is my coworker making my life miserable?" or "My coworker is impossible to work with!"

So now it is your turn to pick one professional and one personal opportunity to define. Give these careful thought because we will use these opportunities for the rest of this chapter in the decision-making process.

Professional opportunity: _____

_____

Personal opportunity: _____

_____

Are they clearly stated and do they have positive outcomes?

 ## Just the Facts

Now it is time to list all the pertinent facts concerning this opportunity. Try to steer clear of opinions. A fact is something that can be shown to be true. Opinions are beliefs based on values and assumptions and may or may not be true.

Now list all the facts that you can come up with concerning each problem. Spend some time on them and then take a break and get away. Allow the opportunity to ferment in your subconscious. Come back again and see if you can add to the lists.

Professional opportunity facts: _____

_____

_____

_____

Personal opportunity facts: _____

_____

_____

_____

Now you are ready to move on to the next step, where you will generate a host of ideas concerning your opportunity for positive change.

 ## Step Two: Generate Ideas Concerning the Opportunity: Seeing the Big Picture

Now is the time to turn on your creative thinking. Remember, quantity of ideas is important at this stage; do not judge or evaluate ideas at this time.

Draw a visual representation of your personal and professional opportunity using associative thinking.

Concept Map

Professional visual representation: Personal visual representation:

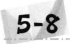 5-8 Tapping into Your Subconscious

The subconscious is a powerful ally in generating ideas about a problem or situation. The subconscious protects us and helps us survive without our even knowing that it is working. This is why many people will have a solution to a problem appear as if by magic when they were not consciously thinking about it. Letting go of a problem allows it to stew in the subconscious, where new ideas and relationships can be established. This activity may seem simple. Try to think about *absolutely nothing* for 3 minutes. Can you do it? It is not as easy as it sounds.

5-9 Letting Go

Choose some type of activity you enjoy. It could be reading, playing a sport, walking in the woods, and so on. Right before you engage in the activity, clearly state your opportunity. Take a couple of slow, deep breaths while visualizing it in your mind. Now do your activity and forget the problem. Immerse yourself in your activity. See if in the next day or two an idea comes to you when you "think" you were not "thinking" about the problem. Careful, you may even dream about it. Write down any ideas that came to you.

_____

_____

_____

_____

_____

_____

5-10 Capitalizing on Peak Creativity

We all have times when we are more creative. For example, some people are most creative on their morning drive to work. They capitalize on this by having a portable cassette recorder ready to record any good ideas that come to them.

1. When are you most creative? _____

2. In what environment are you most creative? _____

3. How do you capitalize on your peak periods of creativity? _____

_____

5-11 Brainstorming Session

Following these guidelines, set up a brainstorming session to further develop ideas concerning your opportunities. If the personal opportunity is too sensitive to share, just do the professional one. However, you are encouraged to do both. Sharing ideas is a great way to enhance your personal growth as an individual.

Guidelines for organizing a brainstorming session are as follows:

• Work in a group of at least three people and no more than eight.

• Choose a comfortable area that is well lighted and free of distractions.

• Assign one person to take notes and record ideas.

• Clearly state the opportunity and the facts concerning it.

• Be spontaneous and imaginative—do not judge or roll your eyes and encourage all to share.

• Listen to other people's ideas and build on them.

- Go for quantity of ideas.
- Do not evaluate someone else's idea.

   1. List the ideas concerning your professional opportunity.

   _____
   _____
   _____
   _____
   _____
   _____

   2. List the ideas concerning your personal opportunity.

   _____
   _____
   _____
   _____
   _____

   3. Jot down some of your impressions of the brainstorming session. What did you like? What did you dislike?

   _____
   _____
   _____
   _____
   _____

 ## 5-12 Step Three of the Decision-Making Process: Evaluate and Select the Best Idea

Now you must evaluate and choose the ideas that are best suited to achieve a positive outcome. For the following exercises, refer to the ideas generated in the previous exercise.

For each idea generated, spend some time visualizing, imagining, and even daydreaming what would happen if you chose and implemented it. After you do this for each idea, list any short- and long-term positive or negative outcomes.

Professional Opportunity

Idea 1:

Short-term positive outcomes:_____

_____

Short-term negative outcomes: _____

_____

Long-term positive outcomes: _____

_____

Long-term negative outcomes:_____

_____

Idea 2:
Short-term positive outcomes:_____

_____

Short-term negative outcomes: _____

_____

Long-term positive outcomes: _____

_____

Long-term negative outcomes:_____

_____

Idea 3:
Short-term positive outcomes:_____

_____

Short-term negative outcomes: _____

_____

Long-term positive outcomes: _____

_____

Long-term negative outcomes:_____

_____

Personal Opportunity
Idea 1:
Short-term positive outcomes:_____

_____

Short-term negative outcomes: _____

_____

Long-term positive outcomes: _____

_____

Long-term negative outcomes:_____

_____

Idea 2:

Short-term positive outcomes:_____

_____

Short-term negative outcomes: _____

_____

Long-term positive outcomes: _____

_____

Long-term negative outcomes:_____

_____

Idea 3:

Short-term positive outcomes:_____

_____

Short-term negative outcomes: _____

_____

Long-term positive outcomes: _____

_____

Long-term negative outcomes:_____

_____

5-13 Step Four: Implementation

If you have more ideas, evaluate them using this same system. Now choose the idea or ideas you think should be implemented. Take at least a few days away from this activity, and then come back and review your work. If you still think you have come up with the best possible solution, move on to the last activity.

Answer the following questions before implementing your solutions.

1. Will implementing this idea have an impact on others? If so, list those people and what type of impact it may have._____

_____

2. What is the best way to communicate this idea to all concerned? _____

_____

3. When is the best time to implement this idea? _____

_____

4. What are the best steps in implementing this solution? _____

_____

5-14 Step Five of the Decision-Making Process: Evaluation

Now implement the solution. After an appropriate period, evaluate its impact and modify it accordingly. Your answers to the following questions will assist you.

1. What positive outcomes should I begin to see?_____

_____

2. When should I see these outcomes?_____

_____

3. Who can give me appropriate feedback?_____

_____

4. How will I know that the solution is working? Be as specific as possible. _____

_____

Do not be afraid to modify your solution when you obtain your feedback. This is normal and occurs often.

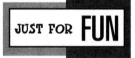

Do Not Be Afraid to Color Outside of the Lines

Connect all the nine dots in Figure 5–5 with four straight lines without lifting your pencil from the paper.

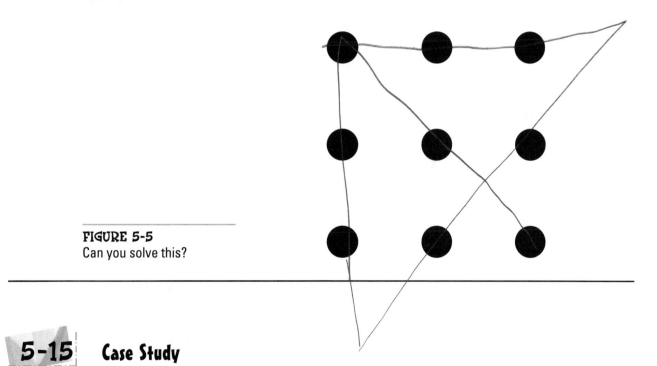

FIGURE 5-5
Can you solve this?

5-15 Case Study

A health care department has decided to implement brainstorming as a method to increase ideas from the employees that can improve communication and morale. During the first brainstorming session, no one was sure exactly what the session was about and there were many distractions of noise and people moving about. During the early part of the session, the supervisor rolled her eyes and let out a heavy sigh when an employee offered up an idea. Very few ideas were generated and little interaction then took place.

Do you think this was a properly run brainstorming session? What do you think actually happened to morale and communication?

_____

_____

_____

_____

Why were there few or no ideas and little interaction during this session?

_____

_____

What could be done to improve the session and make it a positive and productive experience for all?

_____

_____

_____

_____

 5-16 **Internet Activity**

Using Internet search engines, find additional material on thinking and reasoning skills that can help you and your fellow students. Some suggested keywords are: creative thinking, critical thinking, problem solving, reasoning skills, lateral thinking, and decision making. Write down something new that you found to share.

_____

_____

_____

_____

THOUGHTS TO PONDER

> **O**ften, when the conscious forcing of the problem to solution has failed, incubational process succeeds.
>
> - Eugene Raudsepp, Pres., Princeton Creative Research
>
> **W**hy is it I get my best ideas in the morning while I am shaving?
>
> - Albert Einstein

Can you explain why Albert Einstein said this?

SECTION 2

Communicating with Others: Achieving Professional Excellence

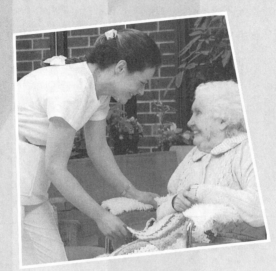

This section discusses communication at an interpersonal level within a group, team, or organization. Basic communication skills are stressed, as is their application to success on the job.

In addition, this section focuses on job-seeking skills. It emphasizes that the time to prepare for gainful employment is *right now!* This is why portfolio development and self-assessment will be a common theme throughout this book. You will analyze and build on your strengths. You will also identify areas that need improvement and create a corresponding action plan.

CHAPTER 6

Types of Communication

OBJECTIVES

Upon completion of this chapter, you should be able to:

List and describe the essential ingredients of the communication process.

Contrast the various types of nonverbal communication.

Explain the various types of verbal communication.

Describe methods to maximize verbal and nonverbal communication.

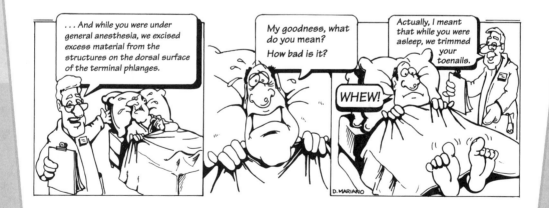

KEY TERMS

communication

communication process

decoding

encoding

enunciation

nonverbal
  communication

oral communication

pronunciation

verbal communication

written communication

INTRODUCTION

The first section of this worktext discusses self-communication. Although this concept is extremely important for your success, you must also learn how to effectively communicate with others. **Communication** for a health care practitioner must occur with patients, family members, and other members of the health care team to deliver safe and effective care. Good communication skills allow health care workers to develop better interpersonal relations with patients, coworkers, and family members. Good communication makes patients feel accepted and helps them develop confidence in the health care professionals who are treating them. Communication helps professionals identify the needs of others and determine how to meet those needs.

But just what is this thing called communication that is so crucial for success? Communication is the exchange of messages, information, thoughts, ideas, and feelings. Communication can be in verbal, nonverbal, or written/electronic form. Verbal communication is primarily the spoken word, such as in conversations, oral reports, voice mail, telephone messages, and speeches. Nonverbal communication includes behavior such as facial expressions, gestures, body language, symbols, and touch. Written and electronic communication include such items as memos, letters, reports, charts, e-mail, and video and computer transfer of information.

THE COMMUNICATION PROCESS

A word is dead when it is said, some say. I say it just begins to live that day.

- Emily Dickinson

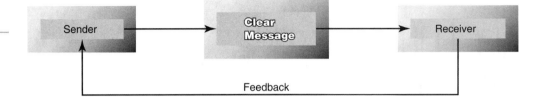

FIGURE 6-1
Basic elements
for effective
communication

If you want a recipe for the effective **communication process**, you must have four basic ingredients: a sender, a clear message, a receiver, and a mechanism for feedback.

Although the process of communication seems simple, it is one of the most difficult tasks that humans perform. The process begins with the sender. The sender is, of course, the person who transmits the message. The sender begins the process by creating a message that he or she wants to convey. The receiver is the person who gets the message. A mechanism for feedback can ensure effective communication because it can confirm that the sender and the receiver have the same understanding of the message that was sent. Figure 6–1 shows the basic elements needed for effective communication.

Let us now take a more in-depth look at this delicate process. The sender is the originator of the idea or message that is to be conveyed. The sender must choose the best way to convert the idea(s) or message(s) into words, diagrams, graphs, reports, and so on. This conversion process is called **encoding** the message. It may be that the sender decides that a memo is the best way to encode a particular thought. In turn, another thought may be best encoded in a personal letter format or sent via e-mail. Each situation must be assessed to determine the most effective way to encode and transfer the thoughts of the sender.

The message that is sent needs to be clearly understood by everyone who receives it. The receiver **decodes** the message, which means that he or she interprets the message. Because messages reach our ears and eyes (body language), it is important that interruptions and distractions be kept at a minimum.

Another important factor in effective communication is making sure that the message is in terms that both the sender and receiver understand. This is especially true for health care workers because we have our own language, called medical terminology. This terminology is often not understood by others not in the health care field.

What Do YOU Think?

Special Considerations When Communicating with Patients

Now that you understand the basics of the communication process, what special considerations need to be taken into account in the health care setting? For example, what about patients who are hard of hearing or heavily medicated? What about patients who can hear but cannot respond because of medication or disease process? Some patients cannot speak because they have a tube inserted through their voice box (larynx) leading into their lungs. What special considerations are appropriate for these individuals? Can you think of any more special circumstances in health care that can impair communication? Refer to Figure 6–2 and identify possible difficulties in communicating with the patient.

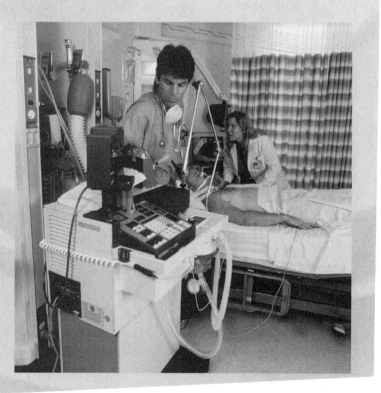

FIGURE 6-2
Can you identify difficulties in communicating with this patient?

You should also avoid slang words or words with double meanings. For example, the word *expire* means to breathe out or exhale. Expire can also mean to die. Therefore, when instructing a patient, it may not be a good idea to say, "I want you to expire now." It would be better to simply say breathe out or exhale. Meaningless terms such as *you know, all that stuff, um,* and *okay* distract from the main message you are trying to convey and should be avoided.

Feedback is an often neglected part of the communication process. The receiver should provide the sender with feedback to show how well the message was received and understood. This can be done in several ways. For example, the receiver can ask questions for clarification, give answers, or react by doing something that demonstrates how well (or poorly) the message was understood. The sender now knows that the message was indeed received and now has some insights about the receiver's interpretation, or decoding.

Once feedback is received, the sender may choose to repeat the message or change the form of the message. In addition, the sender may request further feedback and clarification from the receiver.

Often, patients are the receivers of our messages. Patients may hear messages, but they may not fully understand them because of the unfamiliar terms or just simply because of the environment, which is unfamiliar and sometimes intimidating. Many people do not want to admit that they do not understand terms being used because they think health care workers will perceive them as "dumb." The health care worker should ask questions that require the patient to demonstrate understanding. Simple yes or no questions are not appropriate. The health care practitioner may need to rephrase the explanation until he or she is sure that the patient understands.

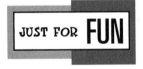

Please Interpret

Listed below are some medical terms. Attempt to explain them to a classmate in lay (everyday) terminology. *Hint:* A medical terminology book or medical dictionary will be of great assistance to you.

Atelectasis

Osteoporosis

Hysterectomy

Rhinitis

Bradycardia

Laparoscopy

Rhinoplasty

Cholecystectomy

 LEARNER:

Go to page 128 and complete the Critical Thinking and Application Activities 6–1, 6–2, 6–3, and 6–4.

TYPES OF COMMUNICATION

NONVERBAL COMMUNICATION

There are three basic types of communication. **Nonverbal communication** consists mainly of body language, whereas **verbal communication** is usually the spoken word; the last form is **written communication**. Our discussion begins with a focus on nonverbal communication.

Nonverbal communication makes up the majority of human communication and may be even more effective than verbal communication. Surprisingly, studies of face-to-face communication show that 80 to 90 percent of the impact of a message comes from nonverbal elements. These elements include facial expressions, eye contact, body language, touch, personal space, and appearance.

Facial Expressions. Many say that a smile is the universal language. The face is a portal that can reflect many of our thoughts and feelings as we are presenting a message. Besides smiles, we can have frowns, scowls, glares, puzzled looks, and so on.

> **N**ature gave you your face, but you have to provide the expression.
>
> - Author Unknown

Eye Contact. Smiles convey a message of friendliness around the world, but eye contact does not. In some cultures, looking downward while speaking is a sign of respect, whereas in the United States, this action may be interpreted as meaning that the messenger has something to hide. However, eye contact is important when talking to patients because it lets them know that you are paying attention.

Body Language. Do you know someone who talks with his or her hands? Do you talk with your hands? We all use body language, whether it is in the form of hands flailing, feet shuffling, finger tapping, head nodding, shoulder shrugging, and so on. Body language can send some powerful signals about how we feel. Body posture is also part of body language. The way you carry yourself while standing or sitting transmits nonverbal messages. For example, someone who maintains his or her body in an upright position with shoulders up and head held high conveys confidence. An individual who walks around slouched over with shoulders and head down conveys a message of sadness and unhappiness.

When interacting with a patient, it is important to lean forward during a conversation to convey the message, "I am interested." If you stand too stiff or tall you may appear tense or uninterested. Crossing your arms also can show an unwillingness to accept what the patient has to say.

Touch. Health care workers use touch to convey compassion and concern. Unfortunately, touch can also take the form of physical and sexual abuse. It is important for health care workers to contrast proper and improper touch. A brief hug, a hand squeeze, or a pat on the back can convey a message of compassion. However, if the touch has any suggestion of sexual or physical abuse it is highly improper. Examples of improper and unacceptable forms of touch include patting, slapping, and stroking of a patient's buttocks or various body parts.

Personal Space or Distance. We also communicate by how little or how much distance we allow between the sender and the receiver. People who know each other well are usually comfortable within a foot of each other. However, to have a complete stranger in your face, so to speak, would most likely make you uncomfortable because he or she has invaded your personal space. People who do not know each other well usually stand 4 to 12 feet apart when they first communicate with each other.

Physical presence, such as bending over someone while trying to communicate, can be intimidating. A patient may perceive this as a stature associated with power and authority and can become intimidated. This is why it is sometimes helpful to sit by the bedside at the patient's level.

Appearance. The way we dress and groom ourselves also sends out powerful messages. Would you have much confidence in a health care practitioner who entered your room in cutoff jeans and a tank top and whose hair obviously had not been washed in days? It makes no difference how competent this individual may be. The nonverbal message that the person cannot care for himself or herself has been sent, and most would interpret this to mean that the person also cannot care for patients. Your appearance has a great effect on your ability to get your message across. Refer to Figure 6–3 and choose the better nonverbal image.

What Do YOU Think?

First Impressions

It may sound corny, but you never get a second chance to make a good first impression. Think about that. If your patients' first impression of you is poor, do you think they will comply with the treatment or have faith in your abilities? Can you think of some examples of nonverbal communication that would enhance a favorable first impression and therefore be the first step in establishing a trusting patient-caregiver relationship. As a start, what about good posture and hygiene? Can you think of more?

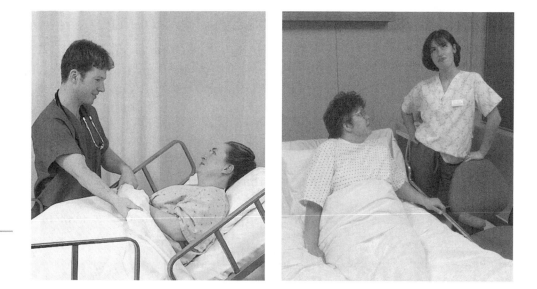

FIGURE 6-3
Which nonverbal
message is better?

Nonverbal Communication

What would the following nonverbal communications mean to you if you were the patient interacting with a health care practitioner who gave these nonverbal messages. Give a brief statement of how you would feel after each gesture.

1. Purposeful silence: _____
2. Handshake: _____
3. Shrug of the shoulder: _____
4. Indirect eye contact: _____
5. Frown: _____
6. Yawn: _____
7. Finger tapping: _____
8. Raised eyebrows: _____
9. One raised eyebrow: _____
10. Pursed lips: _____
11. Facial tension: _____

LEARNER:

Go to page 130 and complete the Critical Thinking and Application Activities 6–5 and 6–6.

VERBAL COMMUNICATION

Instructions and information can be presented to patients, coworkers, and visitors verbally, nonverbally, and even with various audiovisual methods. We have already discussed nonverbal communication, so now we will explore verbal communication in more detail. Verbal communication uses words to convey the message.

In the health care setting, you will use words to explain procedures to your patients and to record and report your observations. Make sure that the terms and concepts that you are presenting are in a language that the listener can understand. You must choose your words carefully so that your message is clear and understandable.

ORAL COMMUNICATION

Oral communication is the form of communication we use often. This is our conversations with our peers, friends, patients, fellow health care professionals, or family members. This form of communication does not always have to be face-to-face. An example would be when you use a telephone or other forms of communication during which you can hear but not see the person on the other end.

Face-to-face discussions provide the best opportunity for the exchange of information, points of view, and instructions, while providing immediate feedback. This feedback can be in the form of return oral communication (questions) or nonverbal cues such as a puzzled look. This can immediately relay signals to the sender that further explanation and clarification is needed.

Several factors enter into the effectiveness of oral communication. These include the manner and tone of your voice, the language used, and nonverbal signals.

Manner and Tone of Voice. The tone and manner of a message can convey excitement, anger, disappointment, cheerfulness, and so on. Your tone of voice reveals your feelings and attitudes. Because tone of voice is so revealing, you should be aware of what you sound like. Remember, it is not always what you say, but how you say it.

The tone, volume, and inflection of your voice can detract from or add to your message. You can either stimulate or calm a patient merely with your voice and behavior. Your voice can have several characteristics, including volume, pitch, and rate.

The volume of your voice refers to its intensity or loudness. In most situations, a moderate volume is appropriate unless the patient has certain characteristics that limit his or her ability to hear you. In addition, when providing a group with patient education, it is more than likely that you will have to raise the volume of your voice for everyone to hear. A good speaker will be able to use volume changes or inflection to emphasize certain parts of the message that he or she believes to be particularly important.

Pitch refers to whether you have a high- or low-pitched voice. People who speak with a high-pitched voice sound shrill and whiny.

Conversely, if your voice is too low pitched, you may be hard to understand. Again, moderation is the key. A moderate pitch with variations is best for standard speech.

Rate is the speed at which you speak. A moderate rate is again best, with some variation so as not to be boring. You can vary your rate by slowing down to emphasize main points or pausing to allow the receiver to reflect on what you said.

Language Used. As a health care professional, you want to be perceived as intelligent, caring, and competent. Your speech can add to or detract from this perception. You should always attempt to speak clearly and concisely and avoid meaningless sounds or message distracters such as *um, uh,* and *okay.*

Everyday, or lay, language is the best when explaining concepts or procedures to patients and family members. For example, say you need to assess a patient's breath sounds. When explaining the procedure to the patient, you should say something such as, "I'm going to listen to how well your lungs sound" versus "I'm going to auscultate your pulmonary system to assess for any adventitious breath sounds." Although the second statement may impress the patient, it will only add distance to establishing trust and communication.

Last, it is also important for you to pronounce words accurately, enunciate (speak clearly), and use good vocabulary and correct grammar.

TEST Yourself

Enunciation versus Pronunciation

Enunciation refers to the clarity with which you say words. Saying *didja* for *did you* or *gimme* for *give me* are examples of poor enunciation. Poor enunciation is the result of leaving out sounds, adding sounds, and/or running sounds together, all of which can confuse patients and may diminish your status among coworkers.

Following is a list of some common terms that are poorly enunciated. Can you identify what the term is? Also, do you properly enunciate the term?

Goin to the pon.

I read the lil pome.

Praps what I said was crul.

C'mere, woodja an gimmee your hand.

Pronunciation is closely related to enunciation. Pronunciation refers to the correctness with which you say words. You are not just running words together or leaving out a letter or two as with enunciation; you are saying the word wrong by mispronouncing it. What is the correct term and pronunciation for the following?

Omost	Famly
Liberry	Burgular
Kindeegarden	Corps
Idear	Jest
Sophmore	Preventative

NONVERBAL SIGNALS

Observation of patients' nonverbal messages will tell you whether they understand or are even listening to your message. This is another reason why it is important to maintain good eye contact with your receiver. As stated earlier, posture can send powerful nonverbal messages along with the conversation. Sitting behind a large desk or in an imposing chair, or standing over the person with whom you are conversing, sends a message that you are powerful and dominant. An environment that contributes to a relaxed atmosphere and has minimal or no outside distractions is most conducive for effective communication. Pay attention to the mannerisms and posture of your patients. These will tell you how they are receiving your verbal message. Are they slouched over, head down, tapping their foot, doodling on paper, and so on?

Finally, listening is a crucial part of oral communication. So much so, that listening is developed more fully in Chapter 7. For now, remember that nothing conveys your interest more in the other person than listening carefully. A conversation is a two-way communication, and you must listen for feedback to make it fully effective. If you monopolize the conversation and do not let others talk, you are also sending the message that what they have to say is not important. Always remember how good it feels when someone is truly listening to you.

LEARNER:

Go to page 130 and complete the Critical Thinking and Application Activities 6–7, 6–8, and 6–9.

WRITTEN COMMUNICATION

In oral communication, no permanent record of what has been said exists. People may forget or even distort part of the message. Although oral communication is used more often, written messages are indispensable and are especially important in health care activities. Written messages are also a more formal means of communication. A well-balanced communication system includes both written and oral communication.

Written communication should be similar to oral communication in that it should be concise and should use understandable language. It is also important that you use proper grammar and ensure that every word is spelled correctly. Diagrams, graphs, drawings, or photographs can be used to show a specific sequence of events or to aid in the understanding of difficult concepts. In addition, films, videotapes, slides, and interactive computer programs can be useful to educate or instruct a patient or family members.

Written messages provide a record that can be accessed and referred to as often as necessary. In addition, written communication can contain better-organized and researched information because you can take the necessary time to organize your thoughts. You can also reread, edit, and redraft your thoughts until you are satisfied with the final document. Written communication is preferred when important details are involved and a permanent record is necessary such as a patient's chart or record.

As a health care professional, you will use written communication often. Some examples are as follows:

- Taking or giving messages and orders
- Writing notes on patients' charts
- Writing policies and procedures
- Developing patient educational material
- Writing memos or letters

What Do YOU Think?

When Does It Need to Be "in Writing"?

Sometimes it is important to follow up an oral conversation or even a confrontation with a written message. A written message may need to follow as a reminder of orally agreed-on duties. For example, if you are a supervisor and request certain tasks of an individual with a certain deadline, you should put this in writing for your sake and the employee's sake.

A written message can also follow an oral communication of a job well done. This way the employee has a positive permanent record to keep on file. Can you think of other instances in which a written message should follow an oral communication?

WRITING A MESSAGE

The first step in writing any message, regardless of its form, is to determine whether it is necessary. Ask yourself, "Can I deliver this message as well if not better by telephone or a face-to-face conversation? Do I need a permanent record of this message for legal or disciplinary actions?"

The second step is to decide what format your message will take. Will it be a letter, e-mail, or memo? Will it be in report form? A memo usually is internal in nature; that is, it stays within the organization. A letter usually is sent outside of an organization. A report can be either internally or externally circulated.

The final step involves the actual writing process. Always consider the five Ws when writing a message:

Who is the primary reader, and who should get copies?

What are you trying to accomplish? What do you want the reader to do? What is fact, and what is opinion? What do the readers already know? What questions are they likely to have? What do you want to avoid?

Why is this important or interesting to the reader?

When will the things happen, and when are the deadlines?

Where will things happen? Where can additional information be obtained?

Figure 6–4 shows the five Ws of a memo.

TEST Yourself

Preparing a First Rough Draft

Your health care club is preparing to do a charity walk to benefit cystic fibrosis. You are in charge of soliciting donations from local businesses. Write a sample letter requesting donations.

Prepare a rough draft using a free flow of thought. This means to simply write as if you are talking. Use your notes on the five Ws and any other critical information that needs to be included. Do not worry about spelling, grammar, and punctuation at this time. Do not worry about your terminology, write the first thought that comes to mind.

Now, review your rough draft, and begin to organize it, trying to keep the reader's perspective in mind. Select an opening statement carefully. This statement is what the reader remembers best, so make sure that it clearly states your main point. Make it an attention grabber by using startling statistics, questions, or something that especially interests the reader.

Rewrite the rest of the message making it short, personal, and to the point. Check each paragraph to make sure that it has a major thought. Each paragraph should flow into the next paragraph and can be linked by words such as *furthermore, consequently,* and *in addition to.*

Prepare your closing statement. This is what the readers remember second best, so it should include some statement about where or whom to contact for further questions or comments, and so on.

Finally, double-check your grammar, spelling, and terminology. You should have no errors in your document. Remember, word processing has good spell-checking programs and a thesaurus to improve the vocabulary. However, when using the thesaurus, remember that although the suggested words may have similar meanings to your original word, they may not have identical meanings. Therefore, it is important that you choose only those words that you fully understand, or you might end up saying something other than what you intended. Also remember that spell checks will not pick up unintended words that are correctly spelled. For example if you type "form" and meant to type "from" the spell checker will recognize form as correctly spelled and not alert you. Always have at least one person read your draft before you send it out.

```
To:      (Whom)  William Smith, Chairperson
From:    (Whom)  Mary Jones, Surgical Technologist
Subject: (Why)   Important meeting
Date:    (When)  October 1, 2006


         (What)  This memo is to inform you of an
                 upcoming organization meeting for
                 the Allied Health Committee.
         (Where) The meeting will take place at the
                 board room of the Administration
                 Building
         (When)  at 10:00 a.m. Nov. 15, 2006.
                 Please RSVP if you can attend.
                 Look forward to seeing you there.
```

FIGURE 6-4
Five Ws of a memo

SUMMARY

Communication is the exchange of messages, information, thoughts, ideas, and feelings. It requires a sender, a clear message, a receiver, and some mechanism for feedback.

Communication can be nonverbal, verbal, or written. Nonverbal communication includes facial expressions, eye contact, body language, touch, personal space, and appearance. Verbal communication includes manner, tone of voice, and the use and selection of language. Written communication provides a permanent record.

LEARNER:

Go to page 132 and complete the Critical Thinking and Application Activities 6–10, 6–11, 6–12, and 6–13.

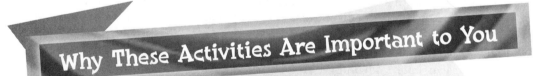

Why These Activities Are Important to You

Communication is an essential part of every aspect of our lives. This includes our personal, school, and future professional careers. Therefore, it is imperative that we learn about the components and types of communication that exist. By learning about the communication process, we can take the first step in becoming effective communicators. Communication is one of the most powerful skills you will ever possess and use.

CRITICAL THINKING AND APPLICATION ACTIVITIES

6-1 One- and Two-Way Communication

This chapter discusses the importance of feedback in the communication process. However, sometimes feedback does not occur because of the pattern of the communication process. For example, in one-way communication, the sender transmits a message, and once the receiver gets it, the process is complete and feedback does not occur. When you receive all that junk mail and simply throw it away, one-way communication has taken place.

List three other examples of one-way communication, either personal or professional.

a. _____

b. _____

c. _____

Two-way communication occurs when the sender transmits a message, the receiver gets it, and there is some type of feedback or response. Conversations are examples of two-way communication, provided that more than one individual does the talking. Of course, if one individual monopolizes the conversation, he or she is probably going to receive nonverbal cues such as rolling of the eyes or tapping of an object or foot as feedback.

List five different examples of two-way communication.

a. _____

b. _____

c. _____

d. _____

e. _____

6-2 Types of Messages

As stated earlier, information or messages can be conveyed by various means. List three examples for each message type, along with an advantage and disadvantage for each.

Example:

Written message: *letter; advantage: can be personal in nature; disadvantage: takes time to send and receive*

Types of Messages

1. a. Written 1: _____

   _____

   b. Written 2: _____

   _____

   c. Written 3: _____

   _____

2. a. Verbal 1: _____

_____

b. Verbal 2: _____

_____

c. Verbal 3: _____

_____

3. a. Nonverbal 1: _____

_____

b. Nonverbal 2: _____

_____

c. Nonverbal 3: _____

_____

6-3 Feedback

Pick a simple procedure to explain to another student. This could be a procedure such as how to properly take a pulse or blood pressure, or it could be some form of patient education concerning a disease process. Record your explanation and interaction, then play it back and evaluate its effectiveness. For example, did you clarify points when they were not understood? Did you use slang or meaningless terminology? Give a written critique of your performances, listing the positive and negative aspects.

1. Positive:_____

_____

_____

_____

2. Negative: _____

_____

_____

_____

6-4 Communication Distortion (The Gossip Game)

Gather a group of at least eight students together in a circle. Have one person start by whispering the following story to the person next to them. Continue doing this until the last person in the group has heard the story. Have this person state the story out loud to the group and then have the first person read the original story. Now compare the results. What did you find? List some of your conclusions.

Story

A patient was brought into the ER with multiple chest trauma from a vehicular accident. The patient was experiencing SOB and had tachycardia with low blood pressure. The patient was rushed to the OR, where a right pneumothorax was found and repaired. He spent two days in the ICU unit and then went to a general care floor. He eventually made a complete recovery and was discharged from the hospital.

Conclusions: _____

_____

_____

_____

 Observing Nonverbal Communication

How much nonverbal communication do you use? Work in groups of three. Designate one person as the observer/recorder. The other two individuals will have a 10-minute conversation, while the observer records (out of their sight) all the nonverbal communication used in the conversation. Switch roles so that everyone gets the chance to be an observer.

Observations: _____

_____

_____

_____

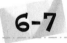 **Mixed Messages**
(When Verbal and Nonverbal Messages Disagree)

Nonverbal communication is said to be more powerful than the spoken words. Have you ever heard someone say, "It wasn't what he said, but how he said it"? Nonverbal communication is difficult to control, and any communication that is not consistent sends a mixed message to the patient. A mixed message occurs when the verbal message is saying one thing and the nonverbal message is saying another, causing a direct conflict.

For example, suppose that a health care professional says, "I'm really excited about the progress in your recovery, you're doing great." However, while saying this, the person had a sad and tense-looking face and the shoulders were slumped forward. Do you think the message was genuine? Would this inspire confidence and trust in that patient?

Have students work in pairs developing a short skit that shows a mixed message. One example could be a therapist and patient in a room where the patient is very concerned about his or her treatment and is asking questions. The therapist *says* that he or she is concerned but frequently checks the times, rolls his or her eyes, taps a foot, or stares out the window.

Describe your skit and the mixed messages: _____

_____

_____

_____

_____

Tone and Manner of Speech

How you say something can greatly change its intended meaning. Working in pairs, practice saying the following statements exactly as they are provided, but vary your tone to convey excitement, disappointment, anger, and so on. See if the receiver can pick the correct emotion.

Statement	Emotion
There is a fire in the room.	_____
You did that procedure well.	_____
I think everything will be all right.	_____
I like talking to you.	_____
Your lab tests turned out well.	_____
No, I don't mind doing that for you.	_____

6-8 Mirroring a Conversation

When you have a conversation, you can mirror the speech and nonverbal actions of your receiver. Mirroring a conversation means that it becomes a reflection of itself. For example, you can match the pace, pitch, tone, volume, posture, or nonverbal messages of the other person. This gives the other person a sense of oneness or connectedness with you, and may help him or her relax and open up to you. Be careful not to mirror everything to the point that it looks like you are mimicking or mocking the individual. The pace of a conversation is usually a good area to control.

For example, if you are talking to someone who speaks very slowly, mirror his or her pace and gradually speed that person up without making him or her aware of it. If you sense that someone is tense, slowly relax your posture and keep your voice calm and facial expressions pleasant. See if this causes the person to relax. You cannot work in pairs with mirroring because the other person cannot be aware of what you are doing. Therefore, practice this technique at home or with friends. Start by seeing if you can alter the pace of the conversation. Experiment and record and share your observations.

Observations: _____

_____

_____

_____

_____

6-9 Self-Assessment

Working in groups of three, have each member do a self-assessment and rate each of the following questions as never, always, or sometimes. Then, pick an observer and have the other two members engage in a 10-minute conversation. The observer will rate the other two on a separate sheet of paper in each of the categories. Use examples as much as possible to justify your ratings. Recording the conversations could be beneficial. Continue until everyone gets a chance to rate the others and compare results.

NOTE: Standard English is the English spoken by news broadcasters, which is free of regional accents. For example, they would not use the western Pennsylvania term *youns,* meaning you all, nor would they speak with a southern drawl and say *y'all.*

1. I speak standard English. _____
2. I speak at a moderate volume. _____
3. I speak at a moderate pitch. _____
4. I speak at a moderate rate. _____
5. I periodically vary my volume, rate, and pitch for emphasis of main points and to maintain interest. _____
6. I use pauses to emphasize major points. _____
7. I enunciate clearly. _____

8. I use proper pronunciations. _____

9. I use appropriate body language and gestures. _____

10. I use correct grammar. _____

6-10 Types of Written Messages

Bring in three different types of short (one to three pages) written communications. Analyze and critique them. What are the positive points? What could make them more effective?

Communication Type 1

1. Positive points: _____

_____

_____

2. Improvements: _____

_____

_____

Communication Type 2

1. Positive points: _____

_____

_____

2. Improvements: _____

_____

_____

Communication Type 3

1. Positive points: _____

_____

_____

2. Improvements: _____

_____

_____

6-11 Writing a Memo

Writing memorandums (memos) is an important aspect of written communication within an organization. Write two memos. One memo should contain an action that needs to be taken, and the other memo should be a description and reminder of an upcoming event. Evaluate your memos using the following criteria and rewrite them if needed. Switch your memos with a partner and evaluate the other's work.

Place a check mark by each of the components your memo contains.

All memos should have a header that contains the following:

To: Include all persons this memo is targeted to reach. Use titles if it is a formal message. Thank-you or congratulatory notes are less formal and may not need titles.

From: The name of the person sending the memo. Again, titles would depend on the formality of the message.

Date: This is the date that the memo was actually sent.

Subject: This statement should be brief and clearly state the main purpose of this memo.

Do your memos contain the proper components of the header? If so, continue.

All memos should have a body or message. Remember, the first statement should hit the main point and grab the reader's attention. The message should contain an action. In other words, is this memo for information only, or is the receiver expected to do something specific? Check and make sure that you have covered the who, what, why, when, and where.

1. Does your memo contain all the components of the message?

2. Does your memo include a closing statement about where or who to contact for further questions or comments?

3. Does your memo have proper grammar, spelling, and terminology?

4. Does each paragraph flow into the next paragraph?

5. Does your memo need to contain attachments such as reference material or reports? If so, these should be noted in the memo and attached.

6. Does your memo need to be copied to others? If so, a list of all parties should be included at the bottom of the memo as follows.

cc: Mr. Smith

Mrs. Jones

Try to limit the memo to one page whenever possible. Use lists, columns, headings, bullets, bolding, and underscoring if needed to organize and make certain points stand out. Some of these techniques (if not overused) also make the memo look impressive.

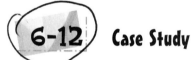 **6-12** **Case Study**

Joliene was about to begin her first clinical experience. She was an above-average student and always did well on her written exams. She studied hard but kept to herself and was very shy. The teacher noticed that she did not make eye contact or smile in class or lab. Joliene always did extra credit and volunteered whenever there were written assignments. Her papers were always outstanding.

What are Joliene's communication strengths?

_____

_____

_____

What are Joliene's communication weaknesses?

She's shy & closed off to peop

_____

_____

Give an action plan that Joliene should utilize prior to attending her clinical rotations in order to make it a positive experience.

_____

_____

_____

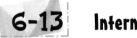 **Internet Activity**

Using Internet search engines, find additional material on types of communication that can help you and your fellow students. Some suggested keywords are: nonverbal communication, oral communication, enunciation, written communication, and writing letters or memos. Write down something new that you found to share.

_____

_____

_____

_____

THOUGHT TO PONDER

Make the most of the best and the least of the worst.
- Robert Louis Stevenson

CHAPTER 7

Communication in Action

OBJECTIVES

Upon completion of this chapter, you should be able to:

Assess environmental and personal barriers to the communication process.

Describe effective methods to break down your defined barriers.

Develop optimal listening skills and use these skills to maximize your communication potential.

Understand the importance of and develop good customer relations skills.

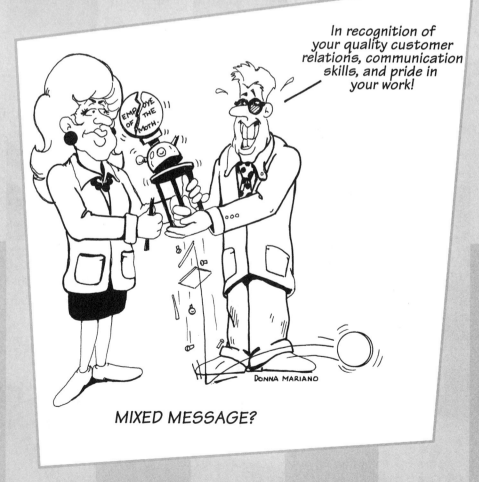

MIXED MESSAGE?

KEY TERMS

active listening
close-ended questions
complacency
customer relations
environmental
   communication barriers

hearing
listening
open-ended questions
personal communication
   barriers
selective comprehension

selective memory
telephone etiquette

INTRODUCTION

Understanding the various types of communications is the first step in becoming an effective communicator. Now we need to look at communication in action in a dynamic system. Are there barriers within us and the environment that inhibit effective communication? Why is listening so important, yet often overlooked in the communication process? Why is effective communications important to an organization? These questions and more are answered in this chapter.

BARRIERS TO COMMUNICATION

Barriers to communication can be either environmental or personal in nature. The environmental barriers include everything outside of the individual that can inhibit communication. For example, excessive noise or poor comfort conditions would impair effective communication. The personal barriers include what is within the individuals who are communicating. These may include emotions, attitude, and prejudices.

ENVIRONMENTAL BARRIERS

The environment can either enhance or detract from the communication process. **Environmental communication barriers** can also be called physical factors.

Noise. If a room is noisy, it will impair your ability to hear as well as the other person's ability. Have you ever heard someone say, "It's so noisy, I can't hear myself think"? Noise levels should be kept at a minimal level. For example, a noisy treatment room can cause not only distraction, but also increased patient anxiety levels.

Activity Levels. If there is a lot of other activity around you, it is easy to become distracted and unable to fully focus on the communication process. Excessive amounts of visual stimulation lessens our ability to fully use our sense of hearing. Have you heard of visually impaired people developing a keener sense of hearing?

Physical Arrangement. How the furniture is arranged can make a difference. Think how you would feel sitting around a small circular table in comfortable chairs communicating with patients. Now picture yourself in front of a large imposing podium on a stage talking down to patients seated in neat rows at hard desks. Which physical arrangement is more conducive for patient education? Physical arrangement should also allow for a private place to talk when needed.

Comfort Levels. If you are physically uncomfortable, it will be difficult for your mental processes to work at peak function. Can you concentrate in a room that is too hot or cold? What if you are uncomfortable sitting or standing while communicating with a patient? Do you think that person may pick up on nonverbal signals showing your discomfort? What if the patient interprets this as a lack of concern? Comfort levels are important for both the receiver and the sender.

Technological Barriers. These can include inadequate telephone capabilities. For example, what if you have excessive static on the line? This would certainly interfere with optimal communication. Another example is using a videotape or DVD for patient education. What if the machine's heads are dirty and the image is poor? Again, this will cause communication to be impaired because of a technological barrier. Computer viruses and errors in e-mail transmissions are becoming more common technological barriers as we increasingly rely on electronic communication.

Time and Distance. An excessive distance between people can act as a barrier. Getting too close and making a patient or coworker uncomfortable can also inhibit communication. The time available to communicate must be adequate to allow for an effective transmission of the message and feedback to occur. Figure 7–1 shows environmental barriers to communication.

PERSONAL BARRIERS

Personal communicational barriers exist within yourself or the person with whom you are communicating. Personal barriers are sometimes not quite as obvious as environmental barriers. Personal barriers can include the following.

Emotional Barriers. Feelings and emotions create barriers to communication. Stress, fear, anger, and sadness can all make it difficult to concentrate on the communication. Positive emotions, such as love and happiness, can also prevent effective communication.

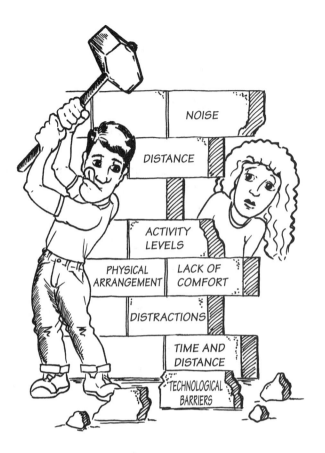

FIGURE 7-1
Environmental barriers to communication

Someone who just won the lottery or found the love of a lifetime may have trouble focusing on ordinary conversations.

Attitudes. Certain attitudes can impair communication. For example, prejudices toward people, because of their religion, race, or membership in a group, is a communication barrier. Racial and ethnic groups are often the targets of prejudice. People can also have negative attitudes toward the elderly, women, men, the poor, the disabled, and people with different lifestyles. You must identify and overcome any type of prejudice that you may have in order to effectively communicate with coworkers and patients who are representative of various groups.

Another type of attitude that acts as a barrier is **selective comprehension**. This is when people focus on the part of the conversation that interests them the most and pay little attention to everything else. Have you ever heard someone say, "You're only hearing what you want to hear"?

Related to this is **selective memory**, when we tend to remember certain things (usually the positive) and forget other things. For example, we may remember and focus on all the procedures we performed well, but we may be "fuzzy" concerning the ones at which we were weak.

Complacency, or indifference, is another attitude that blocks communication. This is the "I don't care attitude." Here, the message may get through, but it is acted on only half-heartedly or not at all.

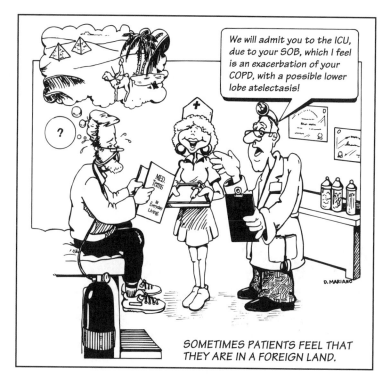

FIGURE 7-2
Use lay terminology!

Language. Words can create a barrier to communication. What if your patient speaks another language? Even if you are both speaking the same language, people do not understand each other for many reasons. For example, often a caregiver will use highly technical language when explaining a technique to a patient. Instead, it is best to use plain, simple words and direct, uncomplicated language that the patient can relate to and understand what you are saying. This is called lay language (Figure 7–2).

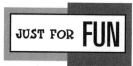

Many Meanings

Many words in our language can have similar meanings depending on how they are used, the tone of voice, and so on. Match the word from List A to a word with a similar meaning in List B. Which list has a negative connotation?

List A		List B
1. E	Firm	**a.** Cocky
2. B	Aggressive	**b.** Ruthless
3. G	Compassionate	**c.** Tactless
4. D	Easygoing	**d.** Unconcerned
5. A	Confident	**e.** Unyielding
6. F	Detail Person	**f.** Picky
7. C	Direct	**g.** Bleeding Heart

Resistance to Change. Have you ever heard someone say, "This is the way we've always done things around here"? Resistance to change is quite common and can be a serious barrier to communication. This is so because many communications may be conveying the message that a new idea, assignment, or change in the daily familiar routine is now warranted. Many people are comfortable with the familiar and prefer things to stay the way they are, which is why it is critical to convey the reason for the change. This will allow people to accept it better.

What Do YOU Think?

Special Patient Circumstances

Patients will often present you with special circumstances. For each of the circumstances described, tell what kind of special communication skills you would use.

1. Patient is confused.
2. Patient speaks a different language.
3. Patient is blind.
4. Patient is hearing impaired.
5. Patient can understand but cannot speak. This is termed aphasia (*a* = without, *phasia* = speech).
6. Patient has just learned that he or she has a terminal illness.

LEARNER:

Go to page 151 and complete the Critical Thinking and Application Activities 7–1, 7–2, and 7–3.

LISTENING

Listening is the often forgotten communication tool. People tend to think of listening and **hearing** as the same thing. Nothing could be farther from the truth. We hear sounds with our ears, but we must listen with our brains. Listening implies paying attention and focusing on the sounds we hear. Listening requires us to concentrate and ignore all the other external and internal distractions. For example, external distractions can be found in a crowded room where we are trying to carry on a conversation. To truly listen, we must drown out all the extraneous noise and focus on the conversation we are part of. Internal distractions include our own mind going 100 miles an hour and not allowing us to focus on anything else.

BARRIERS TO EFFECTIVE LISTENING

Several barriers interfere with our ability to listen effectively. These, like communication barriers, include environmental and personal barriers. Environmental barriers include anything that can interfere with your ability to "hear" the message or any distractions that would interfere with your ability to focus. These include excessive noise levels, uncomfortable environmental conditions, and excessive visual stimulation. Personal barriers include physical and mental characteristics, preconceptions, and self-absorption.

Physical and Mental Characteristics. Listening is both a physical and mental activity. Without being able to hear properly, you lose your ability to effectively listen. The first prerequisite for effective listening is the ability to hear, and this should be assessed for any physiological impairments.

Mental characteristics can affect the ability to listen. If you are not "sharp and focused," your mind will tend to wander to other thoughts. Your physical body is present, but your mind is miles away. The term associated with this phenomena is *daydreaming*. During long, one-sided conversations in which we are not actively involved in the communication process, we may find ourselves daydreaming.

Preconceptions. Have you ever listened to someone and thought, "He doesn't know what he's talking about"? You then have a preconceived idea that what this person has to say is useless, and therefore you will not pay attention. This can be dangerous because then you are not open to other viewpoints that may differ from yours.

Self-Absorption. Have you ever politely listened to someone, while in your mind you were thinking about all the things you had to do? Sometimes we get so caught up in ourselves that it is hard to hear anyone else. This is called self-absorption.

WAYS TO LISTEN EFFECTIVELY

One of the best methods for being an effective listener is to become an active listener as opposed to a passive listener. A passive listener pays just enough attention to keep the conversation going and appear interested. You can usually spot such people by their pleasant nods and frequent "uh-huhs." With these responses, the listener is trying to convince the speaker that he or she is paying attention.

Active listening is a must for important personal and professional communications. Active listening means that your mind is focused on both the message and the speaker. You are attempting to understand the verbal and nonverbal signals being sent your way.

One way to enhance active listening is to ask questions for clarification and to show that you have a curiosity and interest in the message. Another way to ensure that you listen actively is to take notes. Taking notes forces you to pay attention to the message and decide what is important enough to write down.

Another factor that enhances active listening is being open to other views that may conflict with yours. This does not mean that you agree with everything the speaker says, but that you continue to actively listen and not "tune out" the message because you disagree with what it has to say.

Feedback is an important aspect to active listening and probably one of the most effective tools for improving communication. Requiring feedback concerning your message or giving feedback concerning someone else's message is crucial in ensuring that the message is clearly understood.

If you are delivering the message, the simplest way to gain feedback is to observe the receiver and judge the level of understanding. This can be done by looking for nonverbal cues, such as facial expressions. This form of feedback is possible only during face-to-face communication, when you can observe the receiver.

In any type of oral communication, whether it is face-to-face or otherwise, you can get feedback by asking questions or having the receiver repeat the information in his or her own words. Be careful that you ask questions that require more than just a yes or no response.

In general, the most effective questions are **open-ended questions**. Open-ended questions require an explanation as a response. Questions that begin with *what, how,* and *why* are generally open-ended questions. The questions "What do you think we have agreed on?" and "Why do you think you are getting this treatment?" are questions that require elaboration and can relate to you the receiver's level of understanding. **Close-ended questions** are those that can be answered with a simple yes or no. "Did you understand what I just said?" and "Are you feeling okay?" are examples of close-ended questions. To the first question, the feedback may be "yes" even though the patient did not fully understand what you were saying. The reason for this is that some patients may think that they will appear stupid if they say no. Patients may also say "yes" they are feeling well even though they do not because they are in denial and afraid to admit that something is wrong.

Finally, you can get feedback in a written format. For example, you may ask a patient to list the steps that you just explained for performing a procedure at home. This will tell you whether the patient really understands all the steps and the order in which they are to be done. Ways you can improve your listening skills include the following:

1. Avoid barriers such as furniture between you and the other person.

2. Get close to the other person but not so close that you invade the person's personal space and make him or her feel uncomfortable.

3. Sit at the patient's bedside when conversing, versus hovering over the patient, to make him or her feel comfortable.

4. Remain relaxed and friendly, and maintain good eye contact.

5. Do not be distracted by other unimportant events.

6. Have the patient paraphrase what was said to ensure understanding, and ask open-ended questions.

7. Be genuine and sincere. The patient will open up to you and feel more comfortable. He or she will be able to tell whether you are genuinely sincere or just faking interest.

Being a good listener can allow you to establish a positive relationship with your patient (Figure 7–3). Listening will also aid you in gaining valuable information that could assist in the diagnosis and treatment of the patient's condition.

TEST Yourself

How Well Do You Listen?

This is an assessment of your ability to listen effectively. Answer the following questions with this scale:

4 = Always   3 = Often   2 = Seldom   1 = Never

1. _____ I make eye contact with the speaker.

2. _____ I notice the speaker's nonverbal signals (body language).

3. _____ I allow the speaker to finish the complete thought without interruption.

4. _____ I have normal hearing.

5. _____ I ignore other sights and sounds when listening to someone speak.

6. _____ I concentrate on the speaker's thoughts and am not distracted by the way the message is delivered or by the person's appearance.

7. _____ I believe that by listening to other people I can always learn something.

8. _____ If I do not understand something, I ask the speaker to repeat it.

9. _____ I continue to listen even when I disagree with or am uncomfortable with what the speaker is saying.

10. _____ I do not pretend to be listening when I am really daydreaming or thinking about other things.

A score of 30 to 40 means that you are a good listener. A score of 20 to 30 means you can improve your listening skills, especially by focusing in on areas you rated as 1 and 2. A total of less than 20 means you are severely deficient in your listening ability and really need to work on this critical skill.

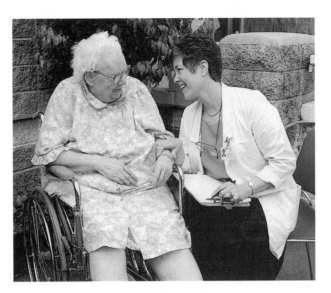

FIGURE 7-3
Listen to your patients.

LEARNER:

Go to page 152 and complete the Critical Thinking and Application Activities 7–4, 7–5, 7–6, and 7–7.

CUSTOMER RELATIONS

Customer relations refers to the way clients (patients and visitors) are treated by the employees of a business. Good customer relations are an essential ingredient in the success of any organization. It is especially important to health care because satisfied customers will return for more services and dissatisfied customers will quickly look elsewhere.

Good communications relate directly to good customer (patient) relations. Many times, choices are made on first impressions. This can often be on the first telephone call made to the health care facility. Proper telephone communication is a must for good customer relationships.

Many health care systems perform public outreach and service in the form of educational seminars and support groups. Therefore, it is important to possess good public speaking skills and understand how to effectively educate patients and their families.

TIPS FOR GOOD CUSTOMER RELATIONS

The following is a list of tips that will optimize good customer relations.

- Learn to recognize steady customers' voices and identify them by name. Recognition means that you value their business.
- Listen carefully.

- Do not make customers repeat themselves. Take notes about the customer's problems or requests. This may include dates and times, order numbers, addresses, and other pertinent information.

- Think critically. You should consider what the customer tells you, eliminate unnecessary information, and pay attention to the heart of the problem or request.

- Do not interrupt. Sometimes customers feel better when they can talk things out. By interrupting, you may break their train of thought, miss crucial information, or increase the customer's anger and frustration.

- Ask questions to help clarify issues and information. Do not ask the same question repeatedly because this usually makes customers think you have not been listening to their responses.

- Solve problems and process requests according to company policy.

- Keep your word. If you say you will call back or take some other action, do it in a timely manner.

- Before terminating a telephone call or personal encounter, ask if there is anything else the person wishes to discuss or if any additional help is needed.

- Follow up. Check with the client later to ensure that everything was done satisfactorily; this shows you value their patronage.

TELEPHONE ETIQUETTE

Your first contact and impression about many organizations occur over the telephone. As has been discussed, you never get a second chance to make a good first impression. Companies realize the importance of good **telephone etiquette** as it relates to favorable customer impressions and satisfaction.

When speaking on the telephone, you lose the nonverbal feedback that is so valuable in effective communications. Until videophones, which allow you to see the other person, are common, you must compensate for the lack of being able to read someone's facial expressions or body language. Therefore, you must focus on your choice of words and voice quality to effectively communicate your message.

Here are some hints on proper telephone use:

- Greeting: Immediately identify yourself and your company or department. For example, "Hello, this is Jane Smith from the radiology department at Acme Hospital. How can I help you?"

- Voice: Talk directly into the mouthpiece, about an inch away, to ensure clarity. Do not eat or drink while talking on the telephone. The annoying sounds can be heard on the other end.

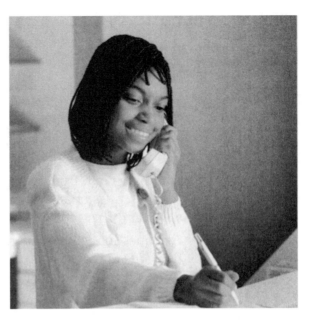

FIGURE 7-4
Your attitude comes
through the telephone.

Speak in a clear and normal volume, and pay particular attention to enunciation. Remember to vary your tone, pitch, and volume for emphasis and to maintain interest.

• Use common courtesy: Be friendly and smile; this will come through in your voice (Figure 7–4). Use the other person's name in your conversation and do not interrupt. If you need to place someone on hold, explain that you will be right back. Be polite. Saying *please* and *thank you* show courtesy, and courtesy shows respect for the caller. When you hang up, gently place the receiver back on the hook; the other person may still be on the line.

• Pay attention: This shows interest. Picture the person on the other end of the telephone, and focus on what is being said.

Always remember that your behavior on the telephone represents the company as well as your personality. How well your company does relates to job security and the potential for your advancement.

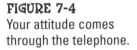

What Do YOU Think?   Customer Relations Assessment

Assess an organization you have had recent contact with in light of the previous reading on customer relations.

1. List three things they did well and give specific examples.

a. _____

b. _____

c. _____

(Continues)

Customer Relations Assessment (Continued)

2. List three areas that need improvement and provide specific examples of how their customer relations can be improved.

a. _____

b. _____

c. _____

3. Finally, how does good customer relations "relate" to individual job security? _____

_____

_____

TECHNOLOGICAL COMMUNICATION

While face-to-face communication may be the mode of choice in most health care situations, technological communication is becoming more prevalent as we advance into the twenty-first century. Communication modes can include fax machines, e-mails, teleconferencing, and text messaging via cell phones. The basic principles of good communication still hold true. Keep the message simple and direct. However, there are some considerations that must be kept in mind as you are composing your electronic message. In most cases, the receiver will not see facial expressions or hear different vocal inflections that may convey added meaning. Therefore, attempt to keep your message as clear as possible and not open to many interpretations. In addition, you must make sure that the message has been properly sent and received because many things can go wrong in cyberspace.

E-mail has gained much popularity as an effective mode of electronic communication because it is:

- Less expensive than mailing a letter
- Usually much faster than the postal service (hence the name snail mail is given to postal mail)
- More conversational in nature
- Less intrusive than a telephone call or fax
- Can readily reach targeted groups of individuals

However, it is not without problems. Make sure that your subject line clearly states the content of the message, or it may be filtered as junk mail and never reach your intended receiver. Double-check your address because one misplaced letter can send it to the wrong person. Also, be very careful when hitting the reply button if the message was sent to a group of people. There have been many cases where a reply was meant only for the sender's eyes but was sent back to the entire group. Do not use e-mail jargon that you use with your friends, and be sure to spell out each word and use correct grammar and punctuation.

Web pages are a very important way an organization can market itself and allow for contact with potential clients. In addition to the jazzy graphics and pictures, Web sites should contain clear and concise information, be easy to navigate, and have contact information such as phone numbers, e-mail addresses, and directions on how to find the organization.

PUBLIC SPEAKING

Health care practitioners are often called on to speak to groups of people. These presentations can be informal or formal in nature and can be presented to patients, families, community groups, or other health care professionals.

The three most important rules for an effective presentation are to (1) be prepared, (2) be prepared, (3) be prepared. Know your subject area well, and organize your presentation in a logical manner that makes sense and is easy to follow. After you have researched your topic well, ask yourself the following questions.

- Who is my audience, and how can I best relate to them?
- What is my audience's interest in the subject?
- Is a formal or informal presentation best?
- What type of supporting materials (handouts) would be beneficial?
- What type of audiovisual material will be most effective for this group?

Think about what type of presenters stimulated your interest most. It was probably people whom you could relate to. It is important to be yourself and let the audience see who you are. Facts and figures are important, but you need to make them relevant to your audience while not overwhelming them. Preparing a simple and logical outline for yourself and your audience will help keep you focused and organized. Remember, people have a difficult time with too much information at once, so keep the presentation simple. Three or four main points are all you need. If you have definitions or graphs, include them on a note-taking outline so that the audience can spend less time writing feverishly and more time listening to what you have to say.

What Do YOU Think?   **Learn from Others**

Think about a favorite teacher or a presentation you attended. What are five characteristics that made a favorable impression on you?

PATIENT COMMUNICATION AND EDUCATION

Communicating with patients is crucial for effective assessment, diagnosis, and treatment. Remember, you are there to provide care and support to the patient. Be open, supportive, and courteous in all your interactions. Listed below are factors to consider for effective patient interaction.

- Answer call bells promptly.
- Focus on the patient's need(s).
- Make sure that you have the patient's attention.
- Speak clearly, using a pleasant tone.
- Use appropriate body language that indicates your interest and concern. Touch the patient, if it seems appropriate. Lean forward, listen to what the patient is saying verbally and nonverbally, and maintain eye contact.
- Allow time for the patient to ask questions.
- Evaluate the patient's verbal and nonverbal responses to assess understanding or treatment effectiveness.
- Ask for feedback in the form of open-ended questions and return demonstrations of procedures.
- Use good listening techniques.

RECORDING AND REPORTING INFORMATION

In health care, an important part of communication is observing or assessing a patient and then recording and reporting this information. You will have to use your sense of sight to observe the patient for color changes, indications of pain, physical abnormalities, levels of distress, and so on. Your sense of smell will help you identify odors that could alert you to certain types of infections. Your sense of touch is critical in feeling for (palpating) a pulse, noting skin warmth, assessing swelling (edema), and performing many therapeutic techniques. Your sense of hearing is needed for listening to the lungs (auscultation), taking a blood pressure, and hearing other normal and abnormal body sounds. Hearing is also needed for effective listening to occur when taking a patient history and identifying the chief complaint. By using all your senses, you can gain a lot of information concerning your patient's condition. The next step is to now record that information properly in the chart and also to give a verbal report to the appropriate persons so the information is correctly passed on (Figure 7–5). Charting and giving reports are covered in an upcoming chapter. For now, just realize it is also an important part of the communication process in giving high-quality care to patients.

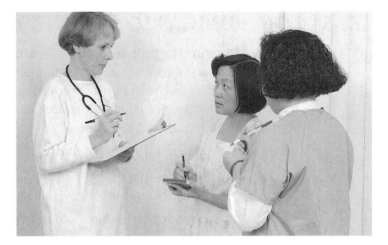

FIGURE 7-5
Recording and reporting patient information is crucial.

SUMMARY

For communication to truly be effective, you must assess and remove the environmental and personal factors that can impair the communication process. An often forgotten part of the communication process is listening. Again, you must break down the barriers that inhibit listening and learn to become an active listener. In a health care organization, patients, families, and visitors all represent customers. Therefore, good customer relation skills must be practiced. Health care practitioners are often needed to do public and patient education and need to enhance their public speaking skills.

LEARNER:

Go to page 153 and complete the Critical Thinking and Application Activities 7–8, 7–9, 7–10, 7–11, and 7–12.

Why These Activities Are Important to You

Understanding the communication process is the first step. You must now put this understanding in action in a dynamic system. Assessing barriers to communication within an individual or organization is a critical action to perform before those barriers can effectively be broken down. In addition, listening is a dynamic aspect of communication, even though it may appear to be a passive process. Finally, good customer relations is essential for any business or organization to continue to survive and thrive.

CRITICAL THINKING AND APPLICATION ACTIVITIES

7-1 Assessing Environmental Barriers

Assess the environmental barriers in your classroom, home, or place of employment. List three barriers with suggested improvements.

Barrier 1:_____

Suggested improvement:_____

_____

Barrier 2:_____

Suggested improvement:_____

_____

Barrier 3:_____

Suggested improvement:_____

_____

7-2 Assessing Personal Barriers

The effective caregiver is aware of and able to identify personal attitudes or prejudices that may interfere with his or her ability to effectively communicate. Once identified, the prejudices can be reduced or even eliminated. This awareness, honest assessment, and the subsequent action to overcome these conditions will make you an excellent communicator.

List two attitudes or prejudices that you have to work on improving. Remember, attitudes can be complacency, procrastination, selective memory, and so on. Prejudices can mean how you feel about the elderly, poor, or people of other races or religions.

Attitude 1: Irritation with people who don't speak english well

Plan for improvement: If I listen closer and have an open mind.

Attitude 2: My own procrastination with projects I'm doing.

Plan for improvement: Besides time management, maybe I could try using a different mind set about getting things done.

7-3 The Language Barrier

Barriers in language that cause poor communication are called semantic barriers. These include using highly technical terms, abbreviations, and jargon. You should always try to be as specific as possible and leave no room for interpretation. For example: "I guess I should" would be better stated as, "I will." "Will one of you take care of this?" would be better stated as, "Mary, please take care of this."

Rewrite the following vague statements.

1. Do you think you could pick me up around six?

   Improved communication: _Please, pick me up at six,_

2. Please make me a few copies.

   Improved communication: _Could you make me a few copies before noon._

3. Do you think you could try to lift this a couple of times?

   Improved communication: _Could you help me lift this a couple of times_

4. I want only a few dollars for my old stethoscope.

   Improved communication: _I want $5 for my old stethoscope_

5. I'm pretty sure you are doing better today.

   Improved communication: _You seem better today, am I correct?_

 Environmental Barriers to Effective Listening

Listening is often neglected or considered to be a passive activity in the communication process. Nothing could be farther from the truth! Listening is one of the most active, dynamic, and effective tools in the communication process.

For one full day, take note of the environmental factors that can act as a barrier to effective listening. Give at least three examples, and explain how the environment can be improved.

Environmental barrier 1: _Too many co-workers working @ once_

Environmental improvement: _Communication was lacking Less coworkers or more organized work space_

Environmental barrier 2: _Trying to skype with my brother but kept loosing connection_

Environmental improvement: _We should have just picked up the phone._

Environmental barrier 3: _While visiting a friend her Phone kept ringing_

Environmental improvement: _Turn all phones & TV off to visit_

 Personal Barriers to Effective Listening

Review the personal barriers for effective listening presented in this chapter. For one full day, take note of any of these personal barriers you observe in yourself or others. List three examples of personal barriers you have observed, and explain how they can be broken down.

Personal barrier 1: _Depression_

Method to break down barrier: _Meds & family support mainly mom, she's my personal cheerleader_

Personal barrier 2: _Lonelyness_

Method to break down barrier: _Make new friends or Surround myself with family_

Personal barrier 3: _Fear_

Method to break down barrier: _Fear of the unknown stuff with John and whats going to happen when all the court dates are done_

7-6 Feedback and Open-Ended Questions

List five open-ended questions you can ask your patient concerning the disease process or the effectiveness of treatment you will be providing.

Question 1:_____

Question 2:_____

Question 3:_____

Question 4:_____

Question 5:_____

7-7 Case Study
The Case of the Inattentive Coworker

You are a night-shift supervisor at a small community hospital. Each night, during report, you distribute and explain staff workloads. One of the employees is always interrupting, chatting about other topics, or just not paying attention. The employee has made a lot of little mistakes in the past and constantly needs to be retold what to do.

1. Why does this employee function poorly? _____

_____

2. What can you do as a supervisor to improve this employee's work performance?_____

_____

7-8 Appreciation of Customer Relations

Good customer relations are crucial for the success of any organization.

1. Pick an organization that you have had recent positive contact with and list three areas of customer relations that impressed you.

   a._____

   b._____

   c._____

2. List three customer relations tips you think would be essential for health care practitioners to use on a daily basis.

   a._____

   b._____

   c._____

7-9 Answering the Telephone

The telephone is often the first contact a customer has with an organization. Each company should have a protocol for answering the telephone. Develop a telephone etiquette policy for a health care department within a hospital. This policy should include protocol for how to handle incoming calls, what to include in the initial greeting, how to take and deliver messages, and who is to handle specific types of calls (e.g., complaints, billing). For example, a part of the policy for the greeting could state that you identify the department, yourself, and your title and then ask, "May I help you?"

Telephone etiquette policy: _____

_____

_____

_____

_____

_____

_____

_____

7-10 Patient Education

Public speaking plays an important role in effective patient education. Develop a 20-minute presentation to a group of patients on one of the following topics:

A group of children, aged 7 to 10 years, on the disease and treatment of asthma

A group of patients with heart disease concerning proper nutrition and exercise

A group of patients with allergies on how to assess and treat the home environment to minimize respiratory problems

A group of diabetic patients concerning proper understanding and treatment of their disease

NOTE: Include objectives, outline, handouts, and method of evaluating the level of understanding of the material you presented.

7-11 Case Study

The health care organization you work for has decided to do more public education programs. You have volunteered to do a program on teaching children and their parents how to better manage their asthma. Your organization feels that a high-quality program will attract more clients and can therefore be greatly beneficial to the organization's health. This could mean a future promotion for your efforts. List three specific actions you can take to ensure that this is indeed a high-quality program.

_____

_____

_____

_____

How will you need to adjust the communication levels for this program?

_____

_____

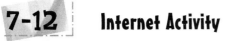

7-12   **Internet Activity**

Using Internet search engines, find additional material on "communication in action" that can help you and your fellow students. Some suggested keywords are: active listening, telephone etiquette, customer relations, communication barriers, and public speaking. Write down something new that you found to share.

_____

_____

_____

_____

THOUGHT TO PONDER

Why do you think people like good listeners? Give three reasons.

a._____

b._____

c._____

CHAPTER 8

Communication Within an Organization

OBJECTIVES

Upon completion of this chapter, you should be able to:

Describe and discuss organizational structure, communication channels, and lines of authority.

Develop an understanding of the factors that affect group dynamics.

Develop optimal group interaction skills and use these skills to maximize your leadership potential.

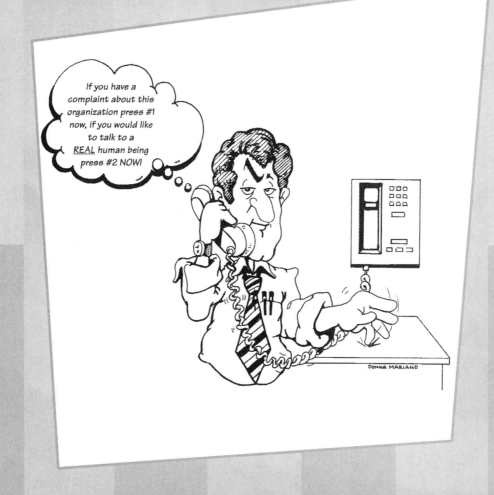

KEY TERMS

cohesiveness
conformity
diagonal communication
downward
   communication
formal communication
   channels
formal groups

gossip
group dynamics
groupthink
horizontal
   communication
informal communication
   channels
informal groups

lateral communication
leadership
norms
organizational chart
rumor
upward communication
vertical communication

INTRODUCTION

> **T**he nice thing about teamwork is that you always have others on your side.
>
>   - Margaret Carty

For any organization to be successful, communication is the number one priority. In health care, communication is essential not just to the success of the organization but also to the outcome of treatments to the patients. Communication must occur within the organization among all health care team members involved in patient care. In addition, various departments in health care organizations must communicate with each other to deliver effective and efficient service for all aspects of the organization. The health care system must also communicate outside the organization to the public, media, and other organizations.

COMMUNICATION NETWORKS

To help employees understand how the organization is put together, an **organizational chart** is developed. This chart succinctly shows many characteristics concerning the organization. The chart shows the flow of communication, the relationships among various departments, and the lines of authority. Figure 8–1 shows a portion of a health care system's organizational chart.

In addition to the organizational chart, every organization has two separate communication channels broken down along formal

157

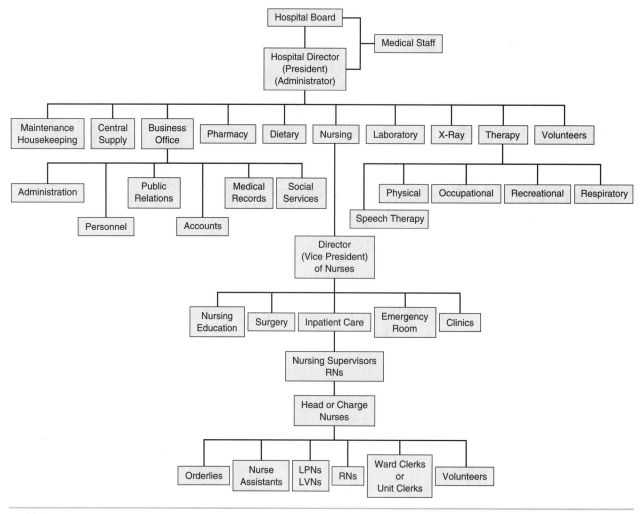

FIGURE 8-1
An example of a health care organizational chart

and informal lines. **Formal communication channels** are established by the way the organization is put together. You can see much of the flow of communication by viewing an organizational structure or flowchart. The **informal communication channels** are sometimes referred to as the "grapevine." Each channel is very powerful and can have a positive or negative effect on the organization's functioning. Formal and informal channels relay messages from one person or group to another in a downward, upward, horizontal, or diagonal direction.

What Do YOU Think?

The Proper Channels

You probably have heard the expression "make sure you go through the proper channels." What does this mean to you? What are the formal channels of communication within your school? What are the informal channels of communication?

DIRECTIONS OF COMMUNICATION FLOW

Information can flow through an organization in a variety of directions. **Downward communication** is a formal flow of communication from people with formal power (managers or supervisors) to staff employees. The flow begins with someone at the top of the structure communicating a message to the next person or group within the hierarchy. This person or persons will then pass it along to those within their group and downward if needed.

Upward communication comes from the staff employees and flows upward to the person or persons in charge. This is as important as downward communication. Be careful not to attach levels of importance to communication channels. All communication is critical, whether it be a directive issued downward from management or a serious problem identified by a staff employee that needs to be brought to a supervisor's attention through upward communication. The supervisor must keep the staff informed, and the employees must feel free to convey opinions and attitudes and to report on the activities of their work.

The combination of upward and downward communication is sometimes called **vertical communication**. Some typical examples of vertical communication are:

- Policies from the management
- Finished products and reports from the staff
- Supervisors' communication with the staff
- Staff communication upward to supervisors
- Written memos, e-mails, letters, and formal reports
- Formal meetings or training sessions

Horizontal communication, or **lateral communication**, is mainly used when departments or groups of people on the same level of the organizational chart need to talk with each other. These may be two departments that are in charge of two different areas where activities overlap. For example, lateral communication often occurs between a nursing floor and the radiological department to schedule procedures. This is important because patients have several other procedures that need to be done, and therefore the nursing department needs to know when to deliver the patient, how long the test will take, and whether there are any special precautions or diets that need to be observed before the test. Horizontal communication is important in facilitating coordination.

Diagonal communication is the flow of communication between departments or people that are on different lateral planes of the organizational chart. For example, nursing personnel may need to contact the housekeeping department when a patient leaves so that the room can be readied for the next patient. To achieve optimal efficiency, effectiveness, and coordination among the various elements of any organization—especially in a health care organization—a free flow of all types of communication (upward, downward, diagonal, and horizontal) is essential.

THE LINES OF AUTHORITY AND RESPONSIBILITY

Someone always has to be in a position to make the final decision or to decide what message is to be sent. The line of authority begins at the top of the organizational chart and can be traced downward throughout the entire organization (Figure 8–2). The line of authority defines the chain of command and establishes the flow of information and responsibility from one individual to another and between departments.

THE GRAPEVINE: THE INFORMAL CHANNEL OF COMMUNICATION

There was a popular song in the 1960s called "I Heard It Through the Grapevine." Unfortunately, as the song illustrates, this is not the best way to hear information. The grapevine may or may not contain factual information. Often, the information contained in the grapevine is based on rumor or gossip. **Rumor** refers to information presented as fact but which has not been officially confirmed. An example of a rumor may be the downsizing of a certain department or division. **Gossip** is more personal in nature and is usually directed at an individual or group of individuals. Some of the characteristics of the grapevine that often make it an undesirable route of communication are:

• Information may be incomplete.

• Information may be based on rumor or gossip and not on facts.

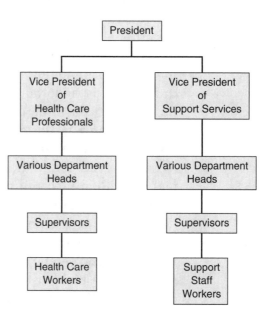

FIGURE 8-2
Lines of authority

- Information may be distorted or exaggerated as it is repeatedly passed on.
- Information may include emotional and prejudicial statements caused by each person's personal feelings.

One way to not become entangled in the grapevine is to avoid office gossip. This will make you stand out as someone who can be trusted with confidential information. Keep what you hear through the grapevine to yourself and do not spread gossip. Stand up for your coworkers when others make unsubstantiated statements about them. This will increase your status within a department as an individual with integrity and one who can be trusted.

What Do YOU Think?

The Office Gossip

You probably know people who gossip a lot. How do you feel about them? Can you trust them with information? Can they maintain confidentiality in the health care setting? Why do people gossip at the office? Have you ever heard of management using the grapevine to disseminate information (especially bad news)?

LEARNER:

Go to page 171 and complete the Critical Thinking and Application Activities 8–1, 8–2, and 8–3.

WORKING WITHIN A GROUP

No matter where you work (unless you isolate yourself from society), you will need to understand how to effectively function within a group. Groups can be either formal or informal in nature. A **formal group** is a collection of people who share clear goals and expectations along with established rules of conduct. As a health care practitioner, your coworkers within your department would represent a formal group of individuals. They would share the common goals associated with quality patient care and the efficient running of the department.

An **informal group** is a loose association of people without stated rules or goals. A group of people at a party or waiting in line for a movie would represent an informal group. Although there are no stated rules in an informal group, there are certain unwritten rules of behavior that are dictated by societal values. For example, skipping ahead in line or starting a fight at a party would be unacceptable behaviors. All groups, whether formal or informal, share certain standards of behavior and characteristic communication patterns that are unique to the group. In other words, people behave differently in groups than they do individually. Understanding these differences will make you an effective group member and enable you to develop team skills that will help you in all areas of your life.

GROUP DYNAMICS

Group dynamics is the study of how people interact in groups. This includes group goals, individual roles, communication patterns, and factors that enhance cohesiveness and positive group interaction. We will now take a more in-depth look at each of these factors.

GROUP GOALS

Just as goals are important for the individual, they are also critical for groups in order to bring focus and direction. Ideally, goals should be developed and agreed on by the group. Just like individual goals, they should be positive and measurable.

Group goals can be cooperative or competitive in nature. Goals are cooperative when the people work together to achieve an objective. A sports team working together to win a game is an example of a cooperative goal. However, competitive goals also exist within the team. For example, each member may be committed to winning as a team but may also have a competitive goal of being the best to get more playing time or to have greater individual recognition.

Most groups have both cooperative and competitive goals. Health care systems in today's environment are organizing their workers into teams or task forces. Members of the team must cooperate with one another to achieve the goals of the team while at the same time possibly competing with other teams in the organization or other outside competitors. Within the team, cooperative goals must be the focus because they enhance communication and productivity. If competitive goals become the major focus, there can be rivalries and secretiveness, which can inhibit communication. However, competitive goals can be a positive stimulus when they create feelings of challenge and excitement and motivate people to do their best.

INDIVIDUAL ROLES

Each person on a team or within a group has a set of expected behavior or responsibilities. These define the individual roles within the group. Roles state what you are expected to do. Within groups, there are certain expectations, or **norms**, by which people in particular roles are expected to adhere.

For example, your role within a health care department may be as a shift supervisor. This job role defines your expected behavior for that position. You may be expected to dole out the work, evaluate employees, mediate conflict, order supplies, and so on. The norms for this position would be someone who is dependable, is hard-working, and has good interpersonal and organizational skills.

In many formal groups, specific roles are assigned to members. For example, a professional organization that represents your chosen health career may have a president, vice president, secretary, and treasurer. In addition, there may be several committees concerning patient care, legislation, communication, membership, and so on. Each committee may have a chairperson whose function is to schedule and run the meeting. A recording secretary may be responsible for recording and distributing the minutes.

COMMUNICATION PATTERNS

Communication within groups can take on various patterns (Figure 8–3). For example, a formal group may have a rigid chain of command that dictates that messages are to be passed down from the top

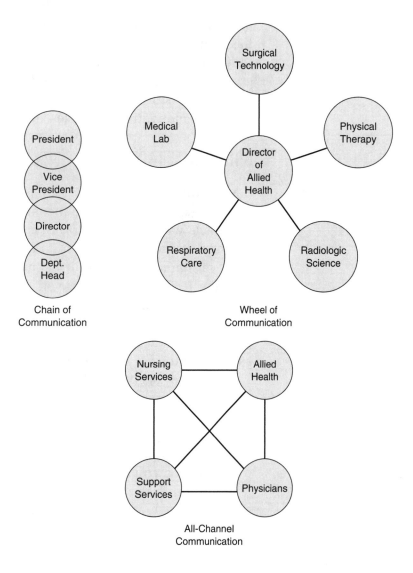

FIGURE 8-3
Various communication patterns of groups

of the organization to the bottom. This can be represented as a chain pattern of communication. Notice how only the links that interconnect are in direct communication.

Another example of a formal communication pattern is called the wheel pattern. Here, one person is the central distributor and controller of the informational flow. An example of this type may be a health care office manager who directs the front desk, billing, nurses, and therapists.

In most organizations, open communication with all members is encouraged. Even in large organizations, tasks and strategic planning are done in smaller less formal groups known as project teams or focused task groups. Here all group members are free to communicate with one another in an open or all-channel pattern of communication. Again, see Figure 8–3, which depicts various group communication patterns.

COHESIVENESS

All groups have various levels of **cohesiveness**. Cohesiveness is measured by the degree to which members work together. Highly cohesive groups tend to have clearly defined roles and goals to which they are strongly committed. Pride and loyalty run high in these groups. Low-cohesive groups tend to be very vague about their goals, and members do not know what is expected of them. Low commitment and motivation characterize low-cohesive groups.

GROUP INTERACTION

Several different interactions that can occur within a group do not tend to occur with individual communications. One such phenomenon deals with group conformity. Changing your opinion or behavior in response to pressure from a group is called **conformity**. Have you ever found yourself doing something just because everyone else is doing it? You may have even done something that went against your personal values or beliefs because you wanted to be accepted as part of the group. It can be very dangerous when an individual gives up his or her values and beliefs and does what the group is doing regardless of the consequences.

Psychologists believe that people who conform to group behavior that is contrary to their beliefs and values have low self-esteem and confidence. In essence, if you conform to the group against your beliefs, the group is thinking for you and deciding what is right and wrong. It is important to act independently when group values contradict your own values.

Conformity is not always a bad thing. In common social group situations, such as a classroom, we conform to the standards by not being disruptive to the educational process. Within a hospital, we conform to the standards of appropriate behavior. For example, a loud and verbally abusive employee is not conforming to the standards of behavior. Here, conformity is good. Remember to be aware when group norms go against your individual values. The important thing about conformity is to know when it is appropriate. Conformity carried to the extreme can lead to **groupthink**. Groupthink is the unquestioning acceptance of the group's beliefs and behaviors. The group becomes the only voice determining what or who is right and wrong. Loyalty to the group becomes more important than anything else. This is a dangerous situation that causes members to lose their ability to think critically and independently. They also compromise their individual values and beliefs. Groups experiencing extreme groupthink can become paranoid and develop an "us against them attitude."

What Do YOU Think?

Groupthink

Can you think of situations in which conformity can be dangerous? What about situations when conformity is appropriate? Can you describe how groupthink can lead to prejudices, hatred, and even wars? Can you give a historical example?

LEARNER:

Go to page 172 and complete the Critical Thinking and Application Activities 8–4 and 8–5.

EFFECTIVE GROUP PARTICIPATION

You can use your knowledge of individual communication techniques coupled with your knowledge about how groups work to optimize your interaction with others. One of the first tasks you should undertake when joining any group is assessment. Group assessment should include understanding and defining group goals and norms. In addition, you should develop a clear understanding of your role within the group. Common questions you should be able to answer for effective group assessment include the following:

• What are the goals of the group?

• Are the group's goals cooperative or competitive (or both)?

• What pattern of communication exists?

• Is this a formal, semiformal, or informal group?

• What is my role within this group?

- What are the other members' roles?
- Does the group have a leader? Who is the leader?
- What are the group norms?

Having assessed the group, your next step is becoming an active participant in the group process. The answers to the preceding questions will help guide your behavior so that you become an accepted, functioning member of the group. For example, if this is a formal group with a set agenda and defined rules of order, you must act in that manner. However, if this is an informal group you can be more casual in your behavior.

Being prepared for the discussion at hand is very important and demonstrates your interest and research capabilities. If you know the agenda or items to be discussed beforehand, you should be prepared to discuss these subjects intelligently. Preparation should include thinking about the subject and reading any relevant or related information.

Using your listening skills will help you become an informed member of the group. Pay attention and keep focused on the subject being discussed. It is beneficial in many situations to take notes, especially if an assignment and deadline are given.

Actively participate by sharing your ideas and respecting the ideas of others, even if you do not agree with them. Be courteous and cooperative with your fellow group members. Take pride in the group and your ability to enhance its functioning.

GROUP LEADERSHIP

Groups need all levels of participants to function effectively, but often a leader is chosen or naturally emerges from within a group. Sometimes the leadership of the group is rotated so that everyone gets a chance. Therefore, it is important that you understand the necessary skills required to lead a group.

Leadership is more than a position or title, it is an attitude and presence. Leadership is a set of behaviors, attitudes, and values that enables the leader to motivate and direct others to act. No matter what is written about leadership techniques, the most effective still is leadership by example.

It is therefore important to develop those qualities that will distinguish you as a leader. Although some people's magnetic or charismatic personalities may make them "born to lead," all of us can learn to become good leaders, even without natural charisma. Most people look for "ordinary but consistent" qualities in a leader that allow them to respect and trust them. Qualities such as the ability to get along with others, good communication skills, trustworthiness, and a strong commitment to goals will make others view you as a potential leader.

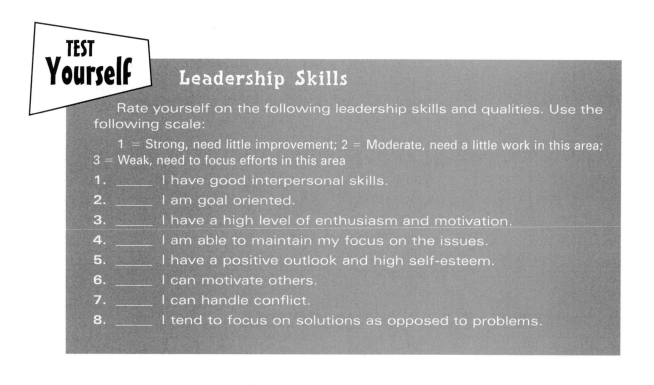

TEST Yourself

Leadership Skills

Rate yourself on the following leadership skills and qualities. Use the following scale:

1 = Strong, need little improvement; 2 = Moderate, need a little work in this area; 3 = Weak, need to focus efforts in this area

1. _____ I have good interpersonal skills.
2. _____ I am goal oriented.
3. _____ I have a high level of enthusiasm and motivation.
4. _____ I am able to maintain my focus on the issues.
5. _____ I have a positive outlook and high self-esteem.
6. _____ I can motivate others.
7. _____ I can handle conflict.
8. _____ I tend to focus on solutions as opposed to problems.

BRAINSTORMING

Another group technique an organization can use to foster creative thinking and generate ideas is brainstorming. Although the term *brainstorming* was coined in the 1950s and has been called several things since, *brainstorming* still says it the best. Group brainstorming is defined as providing an atmosphere in which ideas about any topic, problem, or opportunity can be freely generated. Brainstorming has received attention in business and industry, with much research generated on this process. The literature shows that there are some important criteria for this process to be maximally effective. These include:

- No judgment or evaluation should be made until all the ideas are presented.
- The quantity and *not* the quality of ideas is the major goal.
- Encourage unusual ideas and piggybacking on others' ideas.
- Choose an effective group leader to direct the process.
- Optimal group size is 5 to 8 people

Brainstorming, when done right, promotes progressive employee attitudes that help develop a sense of teamwork and camaraderie. This process helps unclog the communication channels and provides greater mutual respect between individuals and departments.

It is important to do this process right or it can create problems. Some of the pitfalls to avoid in the brainstorming process include a lack of understanding of the brainstorming process and the overselling of the benefits. It will not cure all your problems, but it will generate ideas and increase group cohesiveness if everyone feels free to contribute.

A group leader who can present the problem or opportunity in a positive manner is critical. The leader must not allow any premature criticism, even something as subtle as someone rolling one's eyes. The leader must encourage everyone to contribute. In addition, adequate time should be given for the process to take place. The leader should also provide feedback and praise to the participants and follow up with the results of any of the ideas that may have been implemented as a result of the brainstorming process. Brainstorming can be fun, energetic, motivating, and highly productive if done correctly. However, if done improperly, it can be perceived as a waste of time by the participants. Refer to Chapter 5 for a detailed discussion of brainstorming.

COMMUNICATION AND MEETINGS

Meetings represent another important group interaction that requires good communication skills. Meetings can be held for many reasons. For example, meetings can be used to communicate information, deal with difficult issues, influence attitudes, solve problems, and plan events. Due to the continuing education requirements in health care, often meetings are focused on planning educational programs such as lectures or workshops.

The planning process is critical in ensuring a productive meeting where people feel their attendance was worth their time and effort. The planning process should include who should be invited, the purpose and objectives, and the theme or title of the meeting along with development of a proposed agenda. The location and dates of the meeting should be established as early as possible to reserve the facility and publicize the meeting to the attendees.

As a health care practitioner, you may be required to preside over a meeting. What are some of the things you can do to run a good meeting? First, a warm, personable atmosphere should be established. Refreshments and name tags may be appropriate along with a friendly seating arrangement. At the beginning of the meeting, you should provide a sincere greeting, perform audience introductions if appropriate, and clearly describe the purpose of the meeting. Most meetings are run from an agenda, which lists what is to take place during the meeting. Agendas should minimally include:

- Date and time of meeting
- Location of meeting
- Discussion topics
- Any guest speaker or program if applicable

However, more formal business meetings may require a more standardized agenda and standardized way of running the meeting.

Parliamentary procedure is a set of rules, such as *Robert's Rules of Order,* that help to run larger group meetings and maintain order. In parliamentary procedure, most actions require that a motion be made, seconded, discussed, and then voted on. The motion can be amended (changed) informally if agreement exists with those who made and seconded the motion. Lacking this friendly amendment, a motion can still be made to amend the original motion, but this now needs to be seconded and requires discussion. The amendment is voted upon, after which the main motion is considered again and a vote taken. Did you follow this? This may sound confusing, but after attending a meeting run by these rules, it does make more sense. See Table 8-1 for components of a formal meeting agenda.

Regardless of whether the meeting is formal or informal, the presider of the meeting must be attentive to verbal and nonverbal communication cues. In most meetings, far more is expressed non-verbally than verbally, and presiders can make the meeting more meaningful to more people by being alert to these cues. Are people straining so as to hear or see? Is it too warm or too cold? Is there too much outside distraction? Have people been sitting too long? Is a break needed? Are heads nodding in agreement? Does there seem to be a lot of buzzing about a controversial topic? Is the topic boring, or is it time for a change of format or a change of pace? Is the energy level running low? Are people seemingly anxious to get started on the return trip?

After the meeting concludes, written documentation of what occurred during the meeting must be prepared. This is referred to as the minutes of the meeting. Minutes help to create a history resource for future reference and reminder of decisions made and actions that need to be taken. In addition, minutes serve to inform those who did

TABLE 8-1
Components of a Formal Meeting Agenda

1. Call to order
2. Roll call (if needed)
3. Approval of minutes of previous meeting
4. Treasurer's report
5. Report of officers (if needed)
6. Report of standing committees (if needed)
7. Reports of special committees (if needed)
8. Old business (itemized list)
9. New business (itemized list)
10. Program (if there is a program or speaker)
11. Adjournment

not attend and serve to help form the next meeting's agenda. Minutes should include:

- Date and time of meeting
- Members present, absent, and excused
- Acceptance of previous minutes with any corrections
- Announcements
- Concise reporting of discussions, decisions, and actions that need to be taken
- Date, time, and location of next meeting
- Time of adjournment
- Signature of person preparing the minutes and/or the chairperson

SUMMARY

Communication in an organization can sometimes be confusing. One of the best ways to begin to understand the organization is to review the organizational chart and learn the directions of communication flow. This will also aid you in understanding the lines of authority and where you fit into the big picture. The grapevine is an informal but very powerful part of any organization.

To function effectively within any organization, you must understand group dynamics. This will help you identify the types of groups, group goals, and your role within the group. Many factors (e.g., communication patterns, cohesiveness, group leadership, and groupthink) can affect group functioning. Brainstorming is a great way for groups to generate ideas and begin to interact.

LEARNER:

Go to page 173 and complete the Critical Thinking and Application Activities 8–6, 8–7, 8–8, 8–9, and 8–10.

Why These Activities Are Important to You

You will become part of an organization or team regardless of your chosen health care profession. Even if you are independent and run your own business, the business represents an organization, and you will need to understand organizational communication. In addition, the team concept in organization has gained increased emphasis in the newly emerging health care environment.

Understanding the communication within an organization will keep you connected and informed. This understanding will help you become an integral part of the organization and develop skills that will lead to personal success within the organization.

CRITICAL THINKING AND APPLICATION ACTIVITIES

The Organizational Chart

Pick an organization that you are involved with and obtain and draw its organizational chart. If the chart is extensive, pick a portion that will fit onto this page. You can use your school.

Understanding the Organizational Chart

Understanding the lines of communication within an organization is essential to your success within the organization.

1. From the chart you have drawn, give a description of the informational channels that exist.

   _____

   _____

   _____

   _____

2. Now, identify the following on your chart and briefly describe each:

   Vertical communication channels: _____

   _____

   Horizontal communication channels: _____

   _____

   Diagonal communication channels: _____

   _____

   _____

8-3 The Gossip Game

The grapevine can be a powerful communication tool in the organization. However, it can often distort, exaggerate, or disrupt the communication of the organization. See if the following exercise demonstrates this concept.

1. Form a group of at least 10 individuals. Designate one individual to make up a fictitious story concerning an organization. The story should be at least one typewritten double-spaced page.

2. Form a circle and have this individual whisper the story (reading it exactly as written) into the ear of the person seated next to him or her.

3. Allow the story to be passed on (whispered) to each individual in the circle. Have the last person who receives the story stand up and recite his or her version of the story out loud to the entire group.

4. Finally, have the first individual read the story from the page and compare the results.

Briefly describe the results of this exercise and what it demonstrated to you. _____

_____

_____

_____

8-4 Types of Groups

The understanding of the group process is an important first step in maximizing your ability to work effectively within a team or group of people. Answer the following questions concerning the group process.

1. Identify a formal group that you are a member of. _____

2. List the goals of this group. _____

_____

3. Elaborate on your specific role within this group. _____

_____

4. What type of communication pattern exists? _____

5. How would you characterize the group cohesiveness? _____

_____

6. List factors that are detrimental to group cohesiveness. _____

_____

_____

7. List factors that enhance group cohesiveness. _____

_____

_____

8. Give two examples of informal groups. _____

_____

Conformity and Groupthink

1. Give an example of when conformity to group norms can be dangerous or simply wrong._____
   _____
   _____

2. Give an example of when conformity to group norms is acceptable._____
   _____
   _____

3. Elaborate on an example of when a group is experiencing groupthink. Either use a group you are
   personally familiar with or use a group of people from history._____
   _____
   _____
   _____

4. List the negative outcomes of groupthink to both the group and people outside the group._____
   _____
   _____

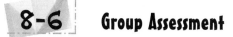 **Group Assessment**

Assess a formal group in which you are a member by answering the following questions:

1. Are the group goals cooperative, competitive, or a mix of both? _____

2. Is the communication formal or casual? _____

3. What are the various roles within this group?_____
   _____

4. What are the group norms?_____
   _____
   _____

5. Who is the group leader? _____

6. How can I maximize my potential within this group?_____
   _____

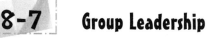 **Group Leadership**

1. From your previous group assessment, list the skills needed to become an effective leader within
   your group. _____
   _____

2. Which of these skills do you already possess? _____
   _____

3. What skills do you need to improve?_____

_____

4. How can you improve your leadership skills?_____

_____

8-8 Brainstorming

Using the guidelines from this chapter, set up small group for brainstorming sessions. Pick a potential opportunity or define a problem about which you would like to generate ideas. Then spend at least 20 minutes brainstorming. Try to schedule at least three separate 20-minute sessions.

1. What were the positive outcomes of the brainstorming session? _____

_____

_____

2. What were the negative outcomes of the brainstorming session?_____

_____

_____

3. How would you improve future brainstorming sessions?_____

_____

_____

8-9 Case Study

You are given the charge to put together a planning committee to develop an educational program for your coworkers on diet and its relationship to diabetes. The objective is to better educate the staff, since they are dealing with an increasing number of patients who have poor dietary habits related to diabetes. List four committee members along with their affiliations or area of expertise. In other words, why would they be effective contributing members of this committee? Remember to bring in as many different perspectives as possible.

Committee member 1_____

Rationale for his or her appointment

_____

_____

Committee member 2_____

Rationale for his or her appointment

_____

_____

Committee member 3_____

Rationale for his or her appointment

_____

_____

Committee member 4_____
Rationale for his or her appointment

_____

_____

Develop an introductory planning meeting agenda for your first meeting.

_____

_____

_____

_____

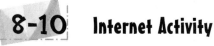 **Internet Activity**

Using Internet search engines, find additional material on communication within an organization that can help you and your fellow students. Some suggested keywords are: communication channels, chain of command, group dynamics, groupthink, brainstorming, and running meetings. Write down something new that you found to share.

_____

_____

THOUGHT TO PONDER

> **W**ork on the same principle as people who train horses. You start with low fences, easily achieved goals, and work up. It's important in management never to ask people to try to accomplish goals they can't accept.
>
> - Ian Mac Gregor

CHAPTER 9

Patient Interaction and Communication

OBJECTIVES

Upon completion of this chapter, you should be able to:

List and explain the four stages involved with effective patient interaction.

Relate the importance of space and territoriality to the patient encounter.

Discuss special issues and concerns when interacting with patients.

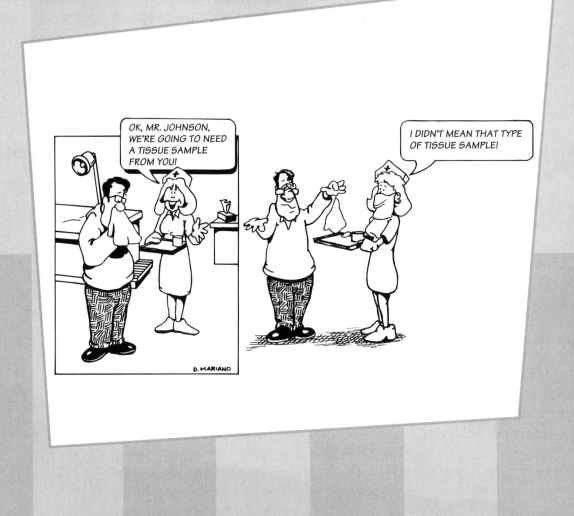

KEY TERMS

charting

chief complaint

intimate space

personal space

social space

territoriality

INTRODUCTION

A faithful friend is a strong defense.
A faithful friend is the medicine of life.

- Apocrypha

There are many procedures that take place before, during, and after each patient encounter. Many thought processes must be performed to near perfection to ensure the safety and comfort of not only the patient but also the practitioner.

All of the previous chapters have prepared you for the initial patient encounter by honing your communication and interpersonal skills. However, a discussion concerning some of the special considerations of communication with patients is needed to complete the picture.

The moment will eventually occur when you walk through a door and there is a patient lying in the room dependent on you. Keep in mind that most patients are not depending on you solely to assess them properly, give them a treatment, or perform other necessary tasks. They are also looking to you as someone to trust and to help them through a difficult time.

This chapter discusses how to effectively interact with patients. Let us begin our journey into one of the most intriguing and rewarding parts of health care—the patient encounter.

PREPARING FOR THE PATIENT ENCOUNTER

Before entering a patient's room, several things must be done. One of the first things a health care worker must do is become familiar with the patient. One of the best places to start is the patient's chart. The chart offers you a plethora of information. The chart is where you will find an almost complete medical history of this person.

You will learn about the patient's reason for seeking medical help. This is often called the patient's **chief complaint** (CC). You will find the patient's name, age, sex, race, and social history (e.g., whether the patient smokes or drinks). You will have a complete medical history and physical to review. Diagnostic tests and treatments are listed with their results. The physician's specific orders are contained in the chart and must be verified before you perform any specific procedure. Take your time with the chart, and get to know a lot about the patient. All this information can facilitate the creation of a bond between the professional and the patient.

TEST Yourself

Medical Lingo

Medical charts contain many medical abbreviations and terminology that represent a unique language. You must be able to understand this language to effectively understand the chart and communicate with others. See how many of the following common terms you know.

STAT _____

MOM _____

bid _____

PRN _____

SOB _____

OOB _____

NKA _____

NPO _____

CPR _____

tid _____

Other things that are important to know and understand are any special precautions that need to be taken. For example, is the patient NPO (nothing by mouth)? This would be very important to know if the patient asked you for a glass of juice. Is the patient allowed out of bed? Must the patient remain flat because of spinal surgery? Should you take any special precautions to prevent the spread of the disease? As stated previously, get to know your patient not only so that you can communicate more effectively with him or her but also so that you can alleviate risks and potentially life-threatening situations.

At this time, you can also talk to other health care practitioners who have interacted with this patient (Figure 9–1). They may be able

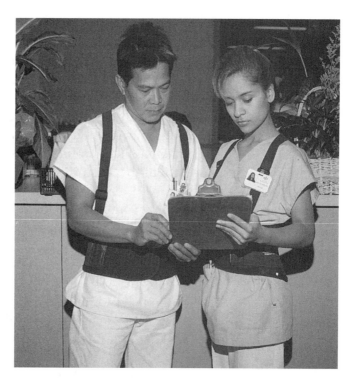

FIGURE 9-1
Review the chart and confer with other professionals concerning your patient.

to give you an idea of the patient's mental state and compliance with treatments. A recent progress note on the chart will also indicate the patient's current status.

THE ACTUAL PATIENT ENCOUNTER

Now that you have learned everything you need to know about your patient, it is time for the initial patient encounter. Sometimes, you are never really prepared for what you are going to find when entering the room, but you handle things as they are brought to you in a professional manner. For example, is your patient going to be in a good mood or bad mood? Is your patient going to be awake or unconscious? Just take things in stride, and do your job well.

At first, you may feel overwhelmed with communicating with your patient while also performing a proper assessment and treatment. This may all seem like too much to remember at once. What do you do first? Take heart in the fact that eventually everything will flow together, and you will develop a routine.

To help you understand the "flow" of events that occur, the patient encounter can be broken down into the following four stages:

1. The introductory stage
2. Patient assessment
3. Treating and monitoring the patient
4. Feedback and follow-up

STAGE 1: THE INTRODUCTORY STAGE

The introductory stage may be considered one of the most vital stages in setting the initial tone of how your patient will perceive you. When you enter the room, the patient may already be wary of you and your intentions. He or she may have been in the hospital for some time now and may be tired of being poked and prodded by different people. This is one reason why it was necessary to research your patient, because it is now time to develop a rapport with your patient.

When you enter the room, formally introduce yourself to your patient and explain who you are and why you are there. For example: "Hello, Mr. Johnson, my name is Tina, and I'm a respiratory therapist. I'm here to give you your breathing treatment this morning." Sometimes you will have patients who are comatose, and you may not see the need for addressing them, but there is a need. These patients are still human and should also be addressed. In time, the patient will get to know you and may allow you to use his or her first name.

The introductory stage is when the patient makes his or her first impression of you. Therefore, it is a good idea to get off to a positive start. If you present yourself in a negative manner or with a false pretense, the patient will sense this. In this situation, the patient may lack trust in your ability to provide treatment. If this happens, things may not go too smoothly the entire time you have this individual as a patient.

You should enter the room in a positive frame of mind. Be friendly but not overly friendly because this may be interpreted as fake. Be professional in the way you act and speak. If a patient asks you a question, answer it to the best of your ability. Another important aspect of patient interaction is eye contact. Do not look out the window when the patient speaks. Look directly at the patient and show that person that you are interested and concerned about his or her thoughts and feelings. Also watch what you say in certain situations. Some patients may be in the hospital for an extended period and may be depressed about their circumstances. You may not help the patient's state of mind if you enter the room and say, "Oh, Mr. Little, it is so beautiful out. The sun is shining, and I can't wait to go golfing." How do you think Mr. Little may feel?

All in all, if you present yourself positively, things will go well; but then again, you will have patients who are difficult to deal with no matter how you present yourself. They may be uninterested in what you have to say or do, and sometimes they may be resistive. Once again, be yourself in these situations and do your job to the utmost. Sometimes you may have to try a little harder with these patients, and they may come around to you.

The number one thing is to show that you care and that you are there because you want to be, not because you have to be. These patients especially need a friendly and professional caregiver to help them through this difficult time in their life.

A friend may well be reckoned the Masterpiece of Nature.

- Ralph Waldo Emerson

What Do YOU Think?

How Would You React?

Often you will develop close relationships with your patients. They may even confide in you with very personal and private information. How would you handle the following situation?

A female pediatric patient has been very withdrawn. However, she has grown close to you and looks forward to her treatment and her interaction with you. You even help her give a treatment to her teddy bear. One day she tells you that she is being sexually abused at home. How would you handle this? What if you got nervous and quickly left the room and avoided the issue? Do you think she would ever develop the courage to tell anyone else?

STAGE 2: PATIENT ASSESSMENT

During patient assessment, you will evaluate the condition of your patient. You will look at the patient's overall appearance, reaction toward you, personality, and attitude. With practice and as your comfort level increases, you will learn how to assess your patient the first moment you walk in the room and begin speaking.

When you assess the patient, you are looking for information that indicates the current health status. This includes inspection of the patient's general appearance and color. Is the patient cyanotic (blue) or jaundiced (yellow-orange)? Is the patient having labored respirations? Does the patient appear confused or anxious? With practice and knowledge, you will soon rival Sherlock Holmes with your inspection skills.

Besides inspection, you may also assess the patient's vital signs, palpate and percuss certain areas, and auscultate the lungs. All the while, you are noting any changes in the patient's physical appearance and watching for any signs of difficulty the patient may be having due to his or her condition. This initial assessment will give you a baseline of data to compare after the treatment. Having this information will help you note changes in the patient's condition. A proper assessment will also aid you in determining whether the treatment prescribed for the patient is appropriate and effective in treating this patient's condition.

STAGE 3: TREATING AND MONITORING THE PATIENT

You have checked the doctor's orders for the prescribed treatment and reviewed the chart. You have introduced yourself, assessed the patient, and determined that the treatment is appropriate and necessary. You also now have a data baseline for this patient before intervening with treatment. Now it is time to actually begin the treatment. While you are administering the treatment, you will need to monitor and assess your patient. Monitoring the patient's vitals throughout the procedure is critical for the patient's safety. If you see any discrepancies from the initial vitals or if the patient seems to be in any distress, stop the procedure immediately and contact the attending nurse and the patient's doctor to communicate the situation.

During the treatment stage, you need to give positive reinforcement and encouragement to your patient. Praise the patient for doing a good job and give assurance that all is going well. Encourage the patient to give his or her best effort during a treatment that requires patient participation. Remember to explain in lay terms why the treatment is being administered and what it will accomplish.

STAGE 4: FEEDBACK AND FOLLOW-UP

Once you have performed all the necessary tasks, it is time to assess the patient one more time. Check the vital signs again, and most important, ask the patient how he or she is feeling. Does the patient feel better, the same, or worse? You are going to want to note all these items on the patient's chart for future reference.

Give your patient specific feedback about how well he or she did with the treatment. Make any appropriate suggestions that would improve the effectiveness of the treatment. Leave with a pleasant, courteous farewell such as, "Thank you, Mrs. Jones, I hope you have a nice afternoon." If you are scheduled to return, let your patient know that you will be back to see him or her.

Now that the patient encounter is over, it is time to record all the procedures that were performed. You will want to chart how the treatment went, how the patient responded to the treatment, the vital signs, the treatment or procedures performed on the patient, and so on. The following is an example of how a respiratory treatment may be charted:

> Aerosol treatment $\times$ 10 minutes with 0.5 cc albuterol and CPT to left upper lobe $\times$ 7 minutes. Breath sounds pre- and post-treatment—rhonchi bilaterally. HR 78–80–79. Patient had good productive cough with moderate amount of thick, yellow mucus. Patient tolerated treatment well. Returned to 3 liter O_2 via nasal cannula.
>
> G. Perry, RRT

Charting is essential to health care. If a malpractice case were to be filed, the chart could be your best friend. It will show the date and time you performed the procedure, and all the therapies performed. This is why it is good to include as much detail as possible and also to assess your patient's status to the fullest.

Each patient has a medical chart which is a legal record that contains biographical data, medical histories, physician orders, physical exam and diagnostic test results, and assessment and progress notes from various health care disciplines. Due to the personal and sometimes sensitive information contained in a chart or during conversations between health care professionals, confidentiality must be maintained. All information given to a health care professional or contained in a chart is considered privileged communication and by law must only be shared with other members of the patient's health care team unless a written consent of permission is given by the patient. There are certain exceptions to this law such as the requirement to report communicable or sexually transmitted diseases and injuries caused by violence that require law enforcement involvement.

Here are some important aspects to charting:

- Always chart the date and time.
- Erasures or whiting out of information in charts is not allowed, and therefore black ink should be used.
- If you make a mistake, place a *single line* through your mistake and write error and your initials above it. (see Figure 9-2)
- Leave no empty spaces when you chart in between notes.
- Charting should be in concise, objective, and accurate language. (Do not interject personal feelings or derogatory statements.)
- Records must be properly destroyed by means such as shredding.
- Abbreviations are allowed if on your organization's approved list.
- Only document what you have done; do not chart for someone else.
- Check for the right patient, the right chart, and that you are using the right form.

Note that most health care facilities use military or international time, not the traditional time used in everyday life. Military time avoids the confusion between AM and PM used in traditional time. For example, if just 4:30 had been written and the AM or PM was omitted,

1. Medicine sheet: *0900 Patient given ▬▬ 100 mg of theophylline orally.*

No adverse reaction noted. M. Johnson R.N.

2. Medicine sheet: *0900 Patient given ~~1000~~ 100 mg Error MJ mg of theophylline orally.*

No adverse reaction noted. M. Johnson R.N.

FIGURE 9-2
Which is legal?

you would not know if this was 4:30 in the morning or afternoon. Military time uses 0100 (1:00 AM traditional time) through 2400 (12:00 AM midnight traditional time). For example, 1630 would represent 4:30 PM. Please see Table 9-1, which shows the conversion between military and traditional time.

Computerized Documentation. With the growing prevalence of computers and computerized charting, additional safeguards must be implemented to prevent others from viewing confidential information. Computer access should be limited to only those health care professionals who should be viewing this information. Using codes and requiring passwords are additional ways to safeguard against unwanted access. Attending orientation training and sessions for any updates to the system will make this process go smoothly. While computerized charting systems do vary, keep in mind to double-check to make sure that you have entered the correct patient identification code, and document or access information only in your authorized areas. Finally, do not share your password with anyone else.

TABLE 9-1
Military (24-Hour Clock) and Traditional Time Conversion Chart

TRADITIONAL TIME MORNING	MILITARY TIME	TRADITIONAL TIME AFTERNOON	MILITARY TIME
12:01 AM	0001	12:01 PM	1201
12:30 AM	0030	12:30 PM	1230
1:00 AM	0100	1:00 PM	1300
2:00 AM	0200	2:00 PM	1400
3:00 AM	0300	3:00 PM	1500
4:00 AM	0400	4:00 PM	1600
5:00 AM	0500	5:00 PM	1700
6:00 AM	0600	6:00 PM	1800
7:00 AM	0700	7:00 PM	1900
8:00 AM	0800	8:00 PM	2000
9:00 AM	0900	9:00 PM	2100
10:00 AM	1000	10:00 PM	2200
11:00 AM	1100	11:00 PM	2300
12:00 noon	1200	12:00 midnight	2400

What Do YOU Think?

The Patient's World

The patient's world becomes the hospital room, especially if he or she has been in the hospital for an extended period. The patient may not be allowed out of bed, and therefore the items on the nightstand (e.g., glasses, tissue) are very important and need to be within reach. Therefore, before leaving the patient's room, put anything you may have moved during the encounter back to where it was.

How do you think the patient would feel if you moved the nightstand before doing the treatment and then forget to return it to within reach? What will this do to your rapport with this patient? What are some other ways that you can respect the patient's world (room)?

LEARNER:

Go to page 191 and complete the Critical Thinking and Application Activities 9–1, 9–2, 9–3, and 9–4.

RESPECTING A PATIENT'S SPACE

Space is a very important aspect of communication that is often overlooked or disregarded in the patient encounter. A patient's room usually becomes a temporary home, and it is necessary for you to respect that patient's territory and individual space. There are three basic categories of space:

- **Social space**
- **Personal space**
- **Intimate space**

Understanding the boundaries and special characteristics of these spaces will enhance your ability to communicate with your patient.

SOCIAL SPACE

Social space is defined as the distance of 4 to 12 feet from the patient. This is where it is most appropriate for you to introduce yourself to the patient and begin the communication process (Figure 9–3). You will be able to see the entire room and patient at this distance and develop a sense of awareness for where everything belongs.

As stated, this is the space for the introductions, but limit what you say because others are in range to hear what you say. Giving confidential or personal information within this space would violate the

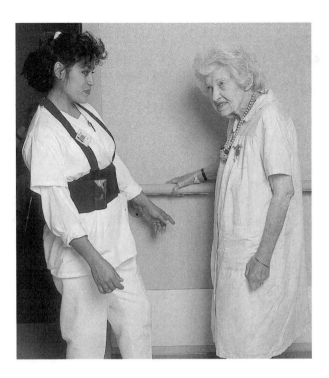

FIGURE 9-3
Social space is 4 to 12 feet from the patient.

patient's trust in your confidentiality. Your approach should be more formal in nature at this point.

PERSONAL SPACE

Personal space is defined as approximately 18 inches to 4 feet between you and the patient. After introducing yourself in the social space, you will move to the personal space, usually at the patient's bedside (Figure 9–4). You are now close enough to the patient at this time to conduct a personal interview without anyone overhearing and at the same time far enough away from the patient so as not to make him or her feel uncomfortable or awkward.

This is the space where you tell the patient about the treatment or ask specific questions concerning the condition. Not only will your body position, manner of speaking, and facial expressions add to the impression, but your general appearance will also. Patients will have more faith in a person who is clean and presentable than in a person who is unkempt and dirty.

This is the space in which you are developing trust with the patient. As stated previously, it is important that communication between you and your patient go smoothly so as to develop trust. Once trust is established, it is easier for you to approach and invade the patient's intimate space, where your assessment and treatment will take place.

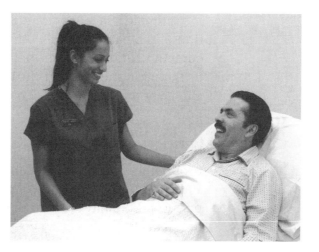

FIGURE 9-4
Personal space is
18 inches to 4 feet away
from the patient.

INTIMATE SPACE

Intimate space is the area about 0 to 18 inches away from the patient. Whereas personal space still allowed patient comfort, invasion of the intimate space can sometimes be awkward for the patient. It is helpful to explain to the patient what you are going to do and why before proceeding with activities in the intimate space. This may improve the patient's comfort level. (Figure 9–5).

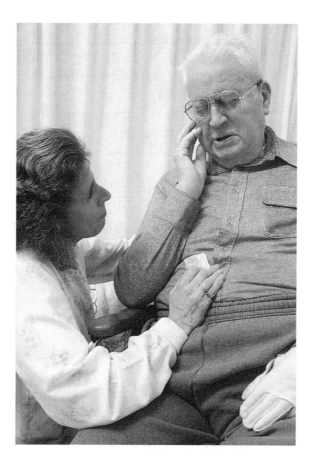

FIGURE 9-5
Intimate space is 0 to 18
inches away from the
patient.

Intimate space is where you will perform the physical examination of the patient. During this period, there is little eye contact and communication between patient and practitioner. Only instruction to the patient is needed during this intimate encounter and performance of the assessment. The instructions should be short and to the point.

The time spent in the patient's intimate space should be relatively short. Perform the physical examination as quickly and appropriately as possible. Many factors, such as the patient's health status, age, and gender, may play a limiting role in the tasks you can perform. You may want to work more slowly and carefully with certain patients.

Respecting the patient's space by beginning in the social and personal spaces and then performing assessments and treatments that invade the intimate space will establish trust with your patient. Can you imagine how you would feel if someone walked into your hospital room and immediately began to take your vital signs or auscultate your lungs without any introductions?

TERRITORIALITY

Territoriality is a major factor in relationships with others. People claim certain space or territory as their own. The patient's room over time becomes his or her turf, or territory. When you enter the patient's room, take notice of where the patient has everything placed. As stated previously, during the treatment, you may have to move things to facilitate the tasks you are performing. Once you finish these tasks, make sure you put everything back where it was. If you move a chair, put it back. Sometimes you may forget, but most likely the next time you see that patient, he or she will say something to you about it.

Putting items back may not be a big deal to you, but it is to the patient. This is the patient's room, and for a lot of patients, it has become home. Patients need to be able to reach things because some may be bedridden. Keep all of these things in mind during patient encounters. Sooner rather than later it will all become second nature.

Territoriality is also important at the nurses' station or medical office. If you remove a chart from a specific area, put it back. For example, charts may be placed in a certain area after a physician writes orders. If you remove a chart from this area for your review and return it to the chart rack, you may seriously delay the implementation of critical procedures or medications.

YOU CAN MAKE A DIFFERENCE

Hope is the pillar that holds up the world.
Hope is a dream of a waking man.
- Pliny the Elder

Many patients you will encounter may have been hospitalized for a long time. Some patients will be comatose; others will be alert and talking. Some will be as pleasant as can be; others will be grumpy and agitated. No matter what type of patient you encounter, you should always treat that person in a professional manner.

Being hospitalized can be one of the most traumatic experiences of a person's life. Many patients become depressed and lose faith. Their life has been turned upside down. They cannot function as they usually would. Sometimes they wake in the morning exhausted because of being awakened at night for medication and treatments. They look forward to having visitors, but sometimes their families and friends cannot make it that day. Some of the patients may have no family at all. These are all factors you must consider. Sometimes you have to think how you would feel if you were that patient. Loneliness and depression can affect the progress of the patient. This is where a health care worker can play a major role in a patient's recovery. Even if the patient's circumstance is terminal, the health care worker can still try to bring a smile to the patient's face. Talk to your patients, check on them throughout the day, see how they are feeling, and see if they need anything. You have already established a rapport, now give them a pillar to lean on, someone to talk to, someone to listen. You will develop many meaningful relationships with your patients that will add to not only their lives, but also your own.

One final but very important note is that health care professionals will encounter various cultural differences in their patient population. It is important to learn about the cultures that exist within your geographical region because this will help you to deliver high-quality care. This will also help you to enrich and improve your own life by appreciating that there are many valid approaches to what someone believes, not only in health care and healing, but also in their views on life.

LEARNER:

Go to page 193 and complete the Critical Thinking and Application Activities 9–5, 9–6, 9–7, 9–8, and 9–9.

SUMMARY

Patient interaction may be the most difficult yet rewarding part of your health care profession. It is important to prepare for your interaction with the patient by assessing the patient's chart and getting all the background information and facts that will facilitate your interaction. The next step is called the introductory stage; during this stage, you introduce yourself and establish a positive impression in the patient's mind. The assessment stage follows, during which you evaluate the patient's condition using the assessment skills that you have mastered. The third stage is the treatment and monitoring stage. It is important to give reinforcement and encouragement during this stage. The final stage is the feedback and follow-up stage, when the patient is told how well he or she is doing with the treatment and the results are recorded in the patient's chart.

Space is an important consideration in treating patients. The three types of space include social, personal, and intimate space. Social space (4 to 12 feet between you and the patient) is for preliminary introductions. Personal space (18 inches to 4 feet between you and the patient) is reserved for the personal interview and discussions. Intimate space (0 to 18 inches between you and the patient) is where you will perform the physical examination and many therapeutic treatments.

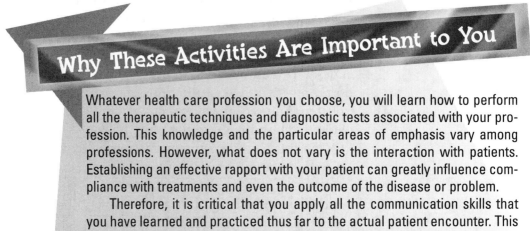

Why These Activities Are Important to You

Whatever health care profession you choose, you will learn how to perform all the therapeutic techniques and diagnostic tests associated with your profession. This knowledge and the particular areas of emphasis vary among professions. However, what does not vary is the interaction with patients. Establishing an effective rapport with your patient can greatly influence compliance with treatments and even the outcome of the disease or problem.

Therefore, it is critical that you apply all the communication skills that you have learned and practiced thus far to the actual patient encounter. This advance preparation and understanding will help your first encounter go much more smoothly than if you had not prepared. However, it may take a while and several patients before you feel totally comfortable with your interaction. This is natural, and we all go through it.

CRITICAL THINKING AND APPLICATION ACTIVITIES

9-1 Preparing to Meet Your Patient

One of the major activities involved in preparation for the patient encounter is reading the chart or medical record. Investigate the makeup and sections of a typical chart at your local hospital. Ask the medical records department to send your class examples if possible. List four distinct sections found in the medical chart, and describe the type of information contained within this section. Have everyone in the class share their findings.

Section: _____

Information contained in this section: _____

_____

_____

_____

Section: _____

Information contained in this section: _____

_____

_____

_____

Section: _____

Information contained in this section: _____

_____

_____

_____

Section: _____

Information contained in this section: _____

_____

_____

_____

9-2 Learning the Lingo

List 10 medical abbreviations and 10 medical terms, and define their meanings. Share the results with the class and develop a large master list.

1. Ten medical abbreviations with definitions:

   a. _____

   b. _____

c. _____

d. _____

e. _____

f. _____

g. _____

h. _____

i. _____

j. _____

2. Ten medical terms with definitions:

a. _____

b. _____

c. _____

d. _____

e. _____

f. _____

g. _____

h. _____

i. _____

j. _____

 Mock Patient Encounters

Work with a partner and pretend that one of you is the patient and one the health care practitioner. Develop a script that has the health care worker go through all the components of the patient encounter, including the introduction, history taking, assessment, vital signs, and a mock treatment. Each group will then perform their skit for the class, and the class will critique the encounter. Each group should have at least one thing done wrong (e.g., forgetting to put the nightstand back) or some unusual characteristic (e.g., a noncompliant patient). See if the class can identify the wrong or unusual circumstance.

 The SOAPIE Note (Not the Halloween Kind)

There is a specific type of nursing progress note called the SOAPIE note. Using your research skills, investigate what a SOAPIE note is and give an example of an actual note.

1. What is a SOAPIE note?

_____

2. Give an example of a SOAPIE note.

S: _____

O: _____

A: _____

P: _____

I: _____

E: _____

9-5 Types of Space

List the three types of space, and give three specific things that should or should not be done within each space.

1. Type of space: _____

Three things that should or should not be done in this space:

a. _____

b. _____

c. _____

2. Type of space: _____

Three things that should or should not be done in this space:

a. _____

b. _____

c. _____

3. Type of space: _____

Three things that should or should not be done in this space:

a. _____

b. _____

c. _____

9-6 Universal Precautions

When you are entering the patient's territory, there are several considerations. One consideration is your not becoming infected by a disease the patient may have. This is why it is important to practice universal precautions. Using your research skills, learn about universal precautions.

Define universal precautions:

_____

_____

_____

Poster Presentation

A poster presentation consists of an organized poster concerning a specific subject. You will be required to explain your poster to the class in a 10- to 15-minute presentation. Your poster will then be put on display. Create a poster presentation concerning one of the following subjects dealing with patient interaction:

- Universal precautions
- Proper handwashing technique
- Aseptic technique
- Proper lifting techniques
- Patient education

9-8 **Case Study**

You are assigned to do quality control for your department. Part of this responsibility is reviewing charts to make sure that proper charting procedures are being followed by staff members. Review the following entry and see if you can identify four mistakes with this charting entry.

Date: 6-24-05 Time 4:30

Patient was given instructions on proper wound care by Mary Beth for 30 60 minutes. Patient wasn't very bright and it took longer than normal to teach the proper procedure.

Charted by Rich Jones

Mistake #1 _____

Mistake #2 _____

Mistake #3 _____

Mistake #4 _____

 Internet Activity

Using Internet search engines, find additional material on patient interaction and communication that can help you and your fellow students. Some suggested keywords are: interviewing patients or clients, medical charting, computerized charting, territoriality, and types of social space. Write down something new that you found to share.

_____

_____

_____

_____

THOUGHT TO PONDER

Courage, love, friendship, compassion, and empathy lift us above the simple beasts and define humanity.

- The Book of Counted Sorrows

Write in your own words what you think this quotation means and how it may pertain to the health professional. Now discuss it in class.

CHAPTER 10

Your First Job as a Health Care Professional

OBJECTIVES

Upon completion of this chapter, you should be able to:

- Perform the steps needed to secure a rewarding career.
- Fully develop the characteristics, attitudes, and interpersonal skills needed to succeed in the workplace.
- Relate the importance of professional image to career success.

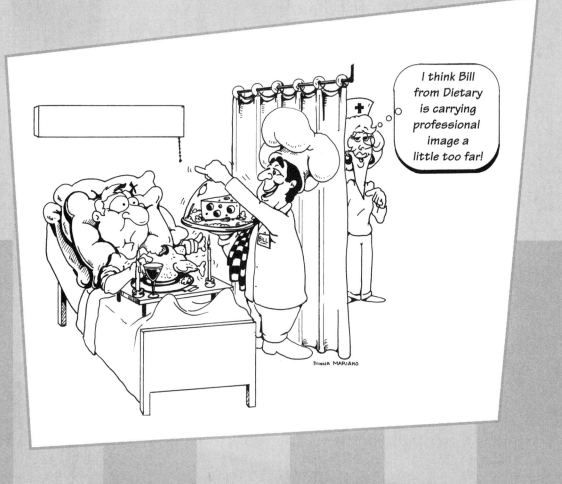

KEY TERMS

cover letter | interview | respect
empathy | professional image | résumé
functional résumé | punctuality | trust

INTRODUCTION

You have worked hard in school to become a health care professional. You have spent hours learning theories, practicing techniques in the lab, doing research, and working with patients. Your hard work will now pay off in the form of your first job as a health care professional.

There are several steps you need to take after graduation to ensure that your first job will be the start of a challenging and personally rewarding lifelong career. These steps include the following:

- Choosing the type of position you wish to secure
- Preparing your résumé
- Making contacts and finding openings
- Making application
- Interviewing
- Accepting a position
- Making a favorable first and lasting impression

This chapter takes an in-depth look at each of these seven steps. Remember, the time and effort you spend on each of these steps will influence the final outcome of the position you receive. Figure 10–1 shows the steps to a rewarding career.

CHOOSING THE RIGHT POSITION

There are several areas of employment and types of positions for a health care professional. For example, you can work in the traditional hospital setting or a rehabilitation unit, or you can perform home care. Opportunities exist in physician offices, outpatient clinics, and surgical units. Skilled nursing facilities and the armed forces offer additional opportunities as do medical and pharmaceutical sales positions. You have to choose an initial job that suits your talents and interests.

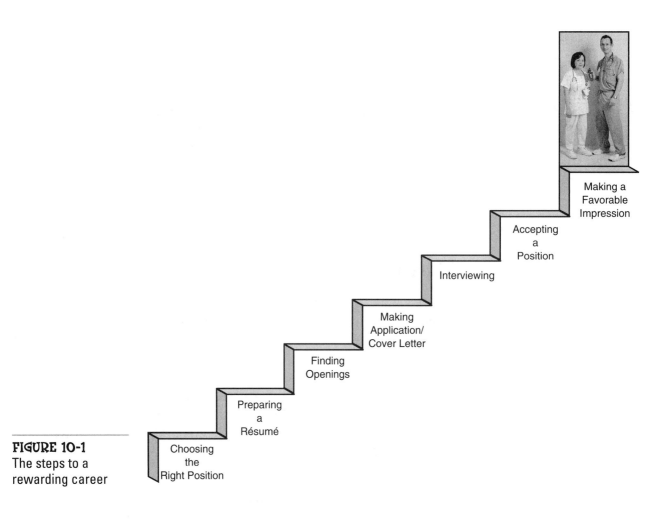

FIGURE 10-1
The steps to a
rewarding career

Taking a careful inventory of your skills, interests, and experience can help you hone in on the right job for you. For example, you may love to work with infants and children. A children's hospital or a neonatal unit may be a place that interests you.

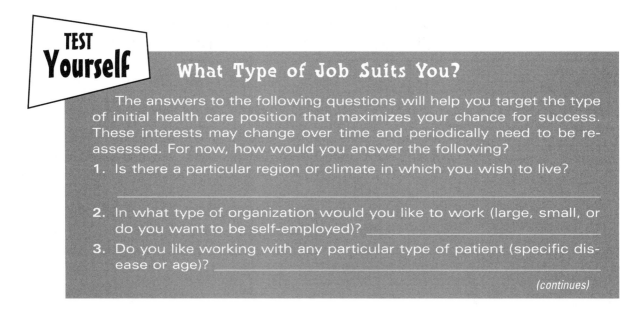

TEST Yourself

What Type of Job Suits You?

The answers to the following questions will help you target the type of initial health care position that maximizes your chance for success. These interests may change over time and periodically need to be reassessed. For now, how would you answer the following?

1. Is there a particular region or climate in which you wish to live?

_____

2. In what type of organization would you like to work (large, small, or do you want to be self-employed)? _____

3. Do you like working with any particular type of patient (specific disease or age)? _____

(continues)

What Type of Job Suits You (Continued)

4. What type of salary range is acceptable to you? _____

5. What benefits are essential to you?_____

6. How important is job security? _____

7. What is it about your profession that really excites you?

_____

Now that you have an idea of what job you want, you are ready to start job hunting. Sometimes in health care, you are fortunate enough to have a position before you graduate. However, this is not always the case, and you can expect to look for weeks or months before finding that ideal position. Do not become discouraged; if you are properly prepared, you will find successful employment. To become properly prepared, a **résumé** is needed.

PREPARING A RÉSUMÉ

A **résumé** is a short summary that highlights "who you are." It tells a potential employer about your education, experience, and qualifications for the job. The résumé is often the first screening tool used by an employer to determine whether the applicant warrants an interview. Therefore, it is essential that your résumé be accurate, complete, neat, and error free. This shows that you took pride in preparing this résumé and are likely to take pride in your work as a potential employee.

Organizing your résumé so that information is easily obtained is important. The information should be kept to one page but not so crowded that it all runs together. Use of white space is important to separate headings.

The information on a résumé is listed in reverse chronological order. For example, your most recent job or degree is listed first, followed by other jobs or degrees in reverse chronological order. As a fresh graduate, you may have little work experience. Therefore, you can develop more of a **functional résumé**. A functional résumé lists your experience in terms of skills you have used on the job or throughout your educational career. To save space, write your information in phrases rather than complete sentences. Get help in preparing your résumé. Ask a knowledgeable person to edit and proofread it. Make sure it is on a computer disk so that it can be easily upgraded and printed out. Use a high-quality printer and paper to produce your final copy.

KELLY CISNEROS
9125 Soledad Avenue
El Paso, TX 79907
(915) 123-4567

OBJECTIVE	Position as a **Back-Office Medical Assistant** in a busy pediatric office
EDUCATION	AS Degree, Medical Assistant, 2000 Caldwell Technical College, El Paso • Perfect Attendance Award three semesters out of four • Grade point average 3.8/4.0 • Externship at Valley Pediatric Center, El Paso • "Excellent Rating" for overall externship performance
EXPERIENCE WITH CHILDREN	6 years providing private daycare in home 3 years teaching disabled preschoolers Cub Scout leader Volunteer tutor at Sanchez Elementary School
ORGANIZATIONAL SKILLS	Maintained state-approved daycare facility Secretary of PTA at children's school Coordinate scheduling and activities for local junior soccer team
COMMUNICATION SKILLS	Make presentations to local organizations about child safety issues Write articles for Sanchez Elementary School parent newsletter 5 years experience as telephone receptionist in a busy insurance office Speak, read, and write Spanish fluently
WORK HISTORY	Cisneros Quality Daycare 1992–1998 Owner of home-based daycare for up to six children SpecialCare Preschool 1989–1992 Teacher Calderon Insurance Agency 1984–1989 Receptionist

FIGURE 10-2
A sample functional résumé

Your résumé should minimally include the following:

- Your name, address, and telephone number
- Your employment objective
- Your education, including school names and addresses, dates you attended, type of program, degree(s) or certificate(s) received
- Your work experience—paid or volunteer (For each job, include job title, name and address of employer, and dates of employment. Your skills can be listed here or in another separate section.)
- Any professional licenses
- Military experience, including branch and length of service, major responsibilities, and special training
- Membership in organizations
- Special skills, foreign languages, honors, awards, and achievements
- An indication that references are available on request

Figure 10–2 shows a sample résumé.

A common and still widely accepted practice is to state "References Available upon Request" at the conclusion of your résumé. However, a recent trend is to omit this statement. If you choose to omit the statement, make sure that you have at least three references with contact information listed on a separate sheet of paper in case they are requested or needed to fill out the job application. Another recent trend is posting your résumé on the Internet or filling out a résumé form electronically online for a specific employer or employment agency.

MAKING CONTACTS AND FINDING OPENINGS

Having prepared a résumé, you are now ready to find job openings that match your employment objective. You can receive information concerning potential jobs from a variety of sources. Some examples of formal sources include the following:

- Classified newspaper ads
- Professional journals and magazine ads
- School placement services
- The Internet
- Job fairs

You can also search by contacting people you know within the health care profession. Many times, they can provide you with inside leads. This informal type of networking is very effective, especially when you extend it to people that your parents, relatives, friends, and fellow students know.

If you have a particular place you desire to work but the organization has no published openings, you should still contact it. Direct contact with a potential employer can provide the organization with a positive impression of your desire and enthusiasm for working there. This will keep you in the employer's mind and give you a possible advantage when the next opening appears. Remember, the more active you are in searching, the more potential opportunities you will identify.

WRITING COVER LETTERS

Now that you have a quality résumé in hand and have identified several potential employers, your next step is to prepare a **cover letter**. The cover letter demonstrates your interest in a particular job and working for a particular employer. Unlike your résumé, which can be copied and sent out to several employers, your cover letter must be specific for each job. Its purpose is to get the employer to want to review your résumé and call you in for an interview. The cover letter should imply that this is "the job" you really want. Major points concerning the cover letter include the following:

- The cover letter should be one page.
- Address the letter to a specific person. Call and find out who that person is versus sending it "To Whom It May Concern." Make sure that you spell the person's name correctly!
- State the purpose of the letter in the first paragraph.
- Elaborate on why your skills and experience match the job.
- Show why you are the person for the job and the value you can add to the organization.
- In summation, ask for an interview and state where and when you can be reached.
- Make the cover letter neat, well organized, error free, and positive.

The cover letter and résumé will get you to the next step in the process—the interview. You may also be requested to fill out an employer application before the interview. Therefore, it is a good idea to bring along a copy of your résumé to serve as a resource when filling out the application. This will demonstrate your preparedness and responsibility. Figure 10–3 shows a sample cover letter.

AD:

DENTAL ASSISTANT. Excellent verbal, scheduling and collection skills. Full-time. Front and back office as needed. Computer literate with good work ethic. Commitment to high-quality patient care.

1357 Keystone Drive
Chicago, IL 60606
July 23,2001

Dr. Harold Mims
1842 Grand Avenue
Chicago, IL 60606

Dear Dr. Mims:

This letter is in response to your ad for a dental assistant. I recently graduated from Harrison Dental College and believe that I fulfill the requirements stated in your ad.

Providing **high-quality patient** care was emphasized throughout the dental assisting program at Harrison. I would welcome the opportunity to begin my dental assisting career in an environment where patients are the top priority.

The program at Harrison emphasized the need for good **verbal skills** in the workplace. We were given many opportunities to practice them. In the skills lab students were required to explain all procedures orally to "patients" before and during hands-on work. I also received grades of "A" in my communication courses, which included Oral Communication and Interpersonal Relations for the Health Care Worker.

I understand the need for a smooth-running **front office** and enjoyed the administrative and **computer training** portion of my training. Performing duties in both the **front and back office** would allow me to apply my organizational skills. My previous jobs, outlined in the enclosed resume, required me to be responsive to the needs of my employers.

My **strong work ethic** is demonstrated in my excellent attendance records, both at school and work, willingness to complete all assigned tasks, and commitment to doing my best at all times.

I would appreciate the opportunity to meet with you to further discuss how I might contribute to the success of your practice. I can be reached at (312) 123-4567.

Thank you for your consideration.

Sincerely,

Kelly Bosner

Kelly Bosner

FIGURE 10-3
Sample cover letter responding to an advertised position

THE INTERVIEW

You have now impressed a future potential employee "on paper." The next step is to see how you interact personally and professionally. The **interview** allows the employer to evaluate your job skills, knowledge, character, and oral communication skills. In essence, the employer is trying to determine whether you are the best employee for the job. The interview is your chance to make a good first impression not only to land the job but also to set the tone for how well you will be received on the job. Therefore, it is critical that you take the time to properly prepare for the interview process.

The interview can be separated into three stages. The preinterview stage is when you learn all you can about your potential job and employer. This is the time to research the organizational goals, vision, and mission statement. You learn about your department and how it fits into the "big picture." You also learn about your job position and what is expected of you. You can call the employee relations or human resources department and request that this information be sent to you, or if it is a local position, you can stop by and pick this information up. Remember to request a job description. Having all this knowledge beforehand will give you added confidence in the interview process.

The preinterview stage can also serve as a practice run-through or stage rehearsal of the actual interview. Here, you can develop answers to questions that are typically asked during the interview process. For example, practice explaining how your skills and experience match the position. The activities at the end of this chapter give you more questions that are often asked so that you can develop a well-thought-out response.

The day of the actual interview has now arrived. A mild level of nervousness and anticipation is to be expected. Your manner of dress and prompt arrival are two very important aspects of the interview process. You should be neat and well groomed with a professional and conservative appearance. Trendy clothes, sneakers, and excessive makeup or jewelry will not impress your potential employer and may even discourage him or her from considering you, no matter how well the interview goes.

Remember to bring a copy of your résumé and a small notepad and pen. The notepad will allow you to take notes and again show your level of preparedness for the interview. In addition, you may want to have some questions prepared in your notepad to ask at the appropriate time during the interview.

Being late for your interview will send a red flag to the employer concerning your professionalism. Make sure you know exactly where the interview is being held, and plan on arriving early. Make sure you have good directions, and if it is someplace you have never been before, you may want to drive out there the day before. Allow for traffic, construction, car problems, or any other unforeseen event.

You can always go to the cafeteria or coffee shop once you know your way to the interview site if you are too early. Plan on arriving at the interview site 10 to 15 minutes early.

While you are waiting to be called in for the interview, make sure you treat the receptionists (and everyone else) with the utmost respect and professionalism. You would be surprised how much of a say they may have in the selection process. When the time has come for the interview and you are called in, remember that you have done your homework and you are prepared. Greet the interviewer(s) with friendliness by introducing yourself and firmly shaking hands. Look each person directly in the eye while speaking to him or her. Wait to be seated until you are shown your chair, as a sign of respect. Let the interviewer(s) initiate the conversation, and follow that person's lead. Everyone interviewing you will be different, and just keep in mind that you are trying to make a good impression as well as learn as much as you can about the job.

Respond to the various interviewers' styles accordingly. Some interviewers may ask very specific questions and expect direct and to-the-point answers. Others may ramble on and want you to do a lot of listening. Still others may ask you open-ended questions such as, "Tell me why you're the person for this job" and expect you to elaborate at length. No matter what the style, you are there to convince them that *you are the best person for the job.* Some "don'ts" of the interview process that can hamper your chance of success include the following:

Top 10 List of Things *Not* to Do at an Interview

1. Don't criticize, complain, or blame others (especially former employers).
2. Don't exhibit nervous or unprofessional habits such as chewing gum, eating candy, or smoking.
3. Don't interrupt.
4. Don't use slang or nonstandard English.
5. Don't discuss controversial topics such as politics or religion.
6. Don't discuss your financial or personal problems.
7. Don't lie.
8. Don't be disrespectful or sarcastic.
9. Don't daydream or lose your focus.
10. Don't forget to be friendly and open and to show your enthusiasm.

Your job is not done after the interview. The postinterview stage is also critical. Here you will follow up appropriately and continue to demonstrate your professionalism as well as your interest in the position. Your follow-up should include a brief thank-you letter for the interviewer's time and consideration. Even if you do not get the position, this will leave a favorable impression for future opportunities. Besides, it is the right thing to do.

Each interview you attend provides you a unique opportunity to critique your performance. What did you do well? In what areas can you improve? Take advantage of each interview as a learning process in sharpening your skills for the future. Do not get discouraged. It may take several interviews to get your first offer. Then again, you may be flooded with offers and have the "nice problem" of choosing the best one.

LEARNER:

Go to page 212 and complete the Critical Thinking and Application Activities 10–1, 10–2, 10–3, 10–4, and 10–5.

YOUR FIRST JOB: FIRST AND LASTING IMPRESSIONS

You never get a second chance to make a good first impression.

- Will Rogers

There are several impressions you want your employer, coworkers, and patients to have concerning your ability to do your job. You want everyone to know that you take pride in your career and that you are a professional. A health care professional has several characteristics, including commitment to quality work, dependability, and a high level of interpersonal skills.

COMMITMENT TO HIGH-QUALITY WORK

The patient represents the consumer of health care services. Although we do not want people to become ill, this is a fact of life. Our job is to prevent and treat illness by providing high-quality services. Quality is important for several reasons. First, the quality of our services directly affects the outcomes of the diagnosis or treatment. Second, the quality of our work increases our individual reputation as well as that of the organization. This in turn results in more repeat and referred customers seeking our services. Without patients, health care systems cannot survive and your position is threatened. In addition, lawsuits can flourish and human life suffer when quality of care is poor. Therefore, it is imperative that you strive for high-quality patient care—for the patient's and the organization's sake.

Quality can best be achieved by doing those things that will make you the best possible health care practitioner you can be. You can be "the best" by learning all you can about your profession. Reading journals, attending seminars, performing continuing medical education, and researching topics will all help you deliver high-quality care because you will be able to use the most current knowledge and techniques.

DEPENDABILITY

Your patients, coworkers, and supervisors need to know that they can count on you to be there. "Being there" in health care can literally mean the difference between life or death. Therefore, it is important to maintain good attendance and punctuality on your job. A good attendance record shows that you are dependable and can be counted on to be there unless a personal emergency or illness occurs. This characteristic allows other members of the health care team to have faith in your commitment. Good attendance also allows for better continuity of care. If members of the team are habitually absent, information is not passed on well and different levels of care may be given.

Punctuality, or being on time at the start of your shift, is especially important in health care. The start of your shift is when the report from the previous shift is given. This report includes vital information concerning your patients' status and their upcoming treatment schedules. In addition, any unusual circumstances or trends can be relayed at this time. For example, it would be highly beneficial to know that the condition of your patient in room 603 is worsening and that the patient had a tachycardia episode during the administration of the last treatment.

Unforeseen things happen in everyone's life, and there comes a time when you will be absent or late. When this occurs, handle the situation in a professional manner. If you know that you are going to be absent or late, make sure your supervisor knows as soon as possible. For example, if you are sick and know you will not make it to work, call as soon as possible (preferably the day before) so that proper arrangements can be made to cover your position. If you are going to be late, again, call as soon as possible and give your approximate time of arrival.

It is also important to be punctual on the job. If you are a member of the trauma or code team, it is vital you arrive ASAP (as soon as possible), or as they say in medicine STAT, when a trauma or code is in progress. In addition, punctuality must be maintained on a patient's treatment schedule. Although this may not always be possible, the patient should be notified when there will be changes in the scheduled treatments or tests.

HIGH LEVEL OF INTERPERSONAL SKILLS

In health care, you must be able to have a positive relationship with your patients and coworkers to deliver effective and high-quality care. This type of relationship can be established by incorporating those attitudes and actions that will lead to a positive outcome. The list of ingredients that leads to a positive relationship include:

- Competency
- Trust
- Empathy
- Respect
- Ability to give and receive feedback

Competency refers to your ability to do your job well. In other words, do you "know your stuff"? This requires you to take pride in your professional career both while in training and after you graduate. You must continue to be a lifelong learner in the health care profession because the advancement of new knowledge and techniques occurs continuously. Competency also requires you to have self-confidence. Even if you "know your stuff," if you doubt your abilities, the patient will perceive you as not competent. In addition, a confident (not arrogant) attitude will be respected by other members of the health care team.

Any good relationship is based on **trust**. Trust means that you can be relied on to get the job done well and maintain professional standards such as ethics and confidentiality. Trust is hard to get but easy to lose. It must be based on consistent behavior that demonstrates that your patients and coworkers can trust you with confidential information.

Respect means that you value your patients and coworkers. Respect is shown by being courteous and understanding in even the most difficult situations. Related to respect is **empathy**. Empathy is the ability to "feel what others are going through." An old phrase states not to judge people until you have "walked a mile in their shoes." Empathy allows us to understand what at times may appear to be irrational behavior.

Positive interpersonal relationships also require feedback to occur. It is important to learn to give and get feedback from your patients and their families as well as from your coworkers. Feedback makes relationships grow and develop. Positive feedback such as praise for a job well done is easy to give and appreciated by the receiver. However, sometimes feedback is negative, which is harder to give and receive.

Feedback should always be given in a nonthreatening manner. The goal of all feedback (even negative) should be to help the other person. Remember, the person who is giving or receiving feedback should always feel respected and valued. General rules concerning feedback include:

- Praise publicly and criticize privately.
- Your motivation with all feedback should be to help the other person.
- Resist judging others when giving feedback.
- Criticize specific behavior and not the individual personally.

TEST Yourself

Do You Have What It Takes?

Picture yourself on the job as a health care practitioner. Drawing from your past work and life experiences, how would you rate yourself in the following areas? Fill in the blanks with *Expert* (no work needed), *Novice* (need improvement), or *Beginner* (need to really work on this area).

1. _____ I am committed to quality and doing the best job I possibly can with every aspect of the job, even the dull and tedious tasks.

2. _____ I am highly dependable and can be counted on to always be there.

3. _____ I am always on time (or even a little early) when reporting for work or meeting with someone.

4. _____ I am constantly learning about my profession and learning new information and techniques to remain highly competent.

5. _____ I can always be trusted with confidential information.

6. _____ I can empathize with others.

7. _____ I respect the rights and beliefs of all individuals, even those I do not agree with.

This is a test in which you should have no *Expert* answers. We can all improve our skills in these areas and should continually strive to do so.

LEARNER:

Go to page 213 and complete the Critical Thinking and Application Activities 10–6 and 10–7.

THE IMPORTANCE OF PROFESSIONAL IMAGE

> **W**e make a living by what we get, but we make a life by what we give.
>
> - Winston Churchill

You are now about to embark on your chosen professional career in health care. Your respective profession is counting on you to represent it in a positive manner to your patients, coworkers, and employer. Joining your professional organization is a very important step in the further development of your **professional image** and career.

Professional image affects the number and quality of persons choosing a certain profession. A high professional image means that more high-quality individuals will choose the profession you represent, which in turn will keep the standards high.

Public opinion is vital to the success of any profession. A positive image affects the outcome of treatments and enhances your interaction with patients. A positive image also lends credence to your interaction with other health care professionals. You can contribute to your professional image by becoming an active member of your professional organization.

METHODS TO IMPROVE PROFESSIONAL IMAGE

The best method for enhancing professional image is to demonstrate that you have the expert knowledge in your field. This can be shown by your competency levels when performing your job, your willingness to learn new procedures, and your continual pursuit of lifelong learning. Reading journals and attending seminars and in-services will lend to this image. The more you know about your profession and your area of expertise, the more difficult it will be to replace you. Therefore, this knowledge relates directly to your job security.

At work always strive to increase your visibility in a positive way. Offer to do in-services and train others both within your department and from other areas. Teaching other health care professionals about your area by providing in-service programs to other departments shows your knowledge, openness, and ability to work as a team member. This helps build camaraderie and mutual respect.

Get involved in health care committees to help network and represent yourself and your profession within the organization. Cooperation with other professionals will maintain an open system of communication and allow your talents to be fully realized. Good luck on your health professional career. You will touch the lives of many people.

SUMMARY

Your first job in health care will be quite rewarding. However, to make sure that you secure the best job for yourself, you must perform several preparatory steps. The first step is analyzing the type of position you want. You will then proceed to develop a professional résumé and make initial contacts and find position openings. A professional cover letter will assist you in getting to the interview stage. Extensive preparation and practice before your interview will enhance your performance and optimize your chance of getting the position.

Once you have secured a position, you must continue to grow and develop in your new profession. You must demonstrate a commitment to high-quality work, dependability, and good interpersonal skills. You must maintain competency by continuing the learning process and maintaining current knowledge about new advances in your chosen practice. Remember to always strive to maintain a high-quality professional image.

LEARNER:

Go to page 214 and complete the Critical Thinking and Application Activities 10–8, 10–9, and 10–10.

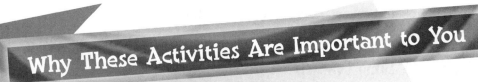

Why These Activities Are Important to You

You have worked hard to graduate from your chosen school and become a professional. However, the work is not done. You must now either decide on more education or look for your first job (in some cases both). Regardless of the path you choose, the potential rewards can be great. These rewards go beyond monetary compensation and include a chance to really make a difference to others' health and lives.

The pursuit of your first job requires careful preparation and planning. This chapter helps you prepare for your quest in finding the position that is right for you. In addition, this chapter conveys the importance of a professional image and lifelong learning. Remember, a health care professional is truly a unique individual. This field requires you to become a lifelong learner in order to maintain competency and stay current within your profession.

CRITICAL THINKING AND APPLICATION ACTIVITIES

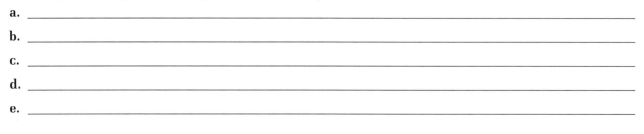

10-1 What Type of Job Do You Desire?

Before looking in earnest for your job, take some time and get a visual picture of just what type of job you desire. Look at your answers to the "Test Yourself" questions in the chapter. Now list the top five attributes of your ideal position. Keep these in mind as you search.

a. _____

b. _____

c. _____

d. _____

e. _____

10-2 Developing Your Résumé

Your résumé is certainly an item that should be included in your portfolio. Remember, your résumé represents you "on paper" to your potential employer. Using what you have learned in this text, coupled with any outside help you can find, complete your résumé. Develop your résumé with word-processing software and save to a disk so that you can periodically update it. Use the following checklist as a review, and check each completed item.

My résumé is:

_____ Neat

_____ Accurate

_____ Well organized

_____ Error free

_____ Comprehensive, containing all the information listed in this chapter

10-3 Making Contacts

List at least five contacts that can help you find a potential job. These can include individuals or classified ads.

a. _____

b. _____

c. _____

d. _____

e. _____

10-4 The Cover Letter

Again, using what you have learned from your text and outside sources, develop a cover letter to one of the contacts mentioned in the previous activity.

10-5 The Interview

Working together in a small group, take turns being the interviewer and the interviewee. Have a third student critique the interviewee or, if possible, videotape the interview process and let everyone critique the performance. Videotaping and viewing yourself perform can identify weak areas such as nervous habits that you may not even be aware you do.

List five areas you will work on to improve from your evaluations of your interview process.

a. _____

b. _____

c. _____

d. _____

e. _____

10-6 Impressions on the Job

For each word or phrase listed, give a brief explanation of what it means to you personally. Then, write a sentence on how it will relate to you in your first job in health care.

1. Commitment to quality work
   Personal meaning:_____
   How does it relate to my first job in health care? _____

   _____

2. Dependability
   Personal meaning:_____
   How does it relate to my first job in health care? _____

   _____

3. Punctuality
   Personal meaning:_____
   How does it relate to my first job in health care? _____

   _____

4. Empathy
   Personal meaning:_____
   How does it relate to my first job in health care? _____

   _____

5. Trust
   Personal meaning:_____
   How does it relate to my first job in health care? _____

   _____

6. Respect
   Personal meaning:_____
   How does it relate to my first job in health care? _____

   _____

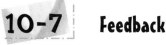 Feedback

1. Give an example of when you handled negative feedback appropriately. _____
   _____
   _____

2. Give an example of when you did not handle feedback appropriately. _____
   _____
   _____

Investigating Your Profession

Learning about your chosen profession is the first important step in achieving a high professional image. Call the national headquarters for your profession and obtain as much information as you can to answer the following:

1. Name of profession: _____

2. Headquarters' address and telephone numbers: _____
   _____

3. Profession description: _____
   _____
   _____
   _____

4. Professional credentials: _____
   _____
   _____

5. Professional publications: _____
   _____

10-9 Case Study

Tara Smith worked as a dental technician in the office for almost 4 years. Tara was a dependable employee and performed adequately with good technical skills. She made no effort to "go above and beyond the call" and did not keep up with advances in her field by attending seminars or conferences or volunteer for special projects. She was never rude to her clients but gave the impression she was simply doing her job and anxious to finish her shift. Tara was very surprised and upset when a coworker who was only in the office for a little over a year got a promotion she thought she had deserved. Is Tara's disappointment justified? Describe some of the things she could have done differently in order to put herself in a better position to get future promotions.

_____
_____
_____
_____

10-10 Internet Activity

Using Internet search engines, find additional material on "your first job as a health care professional" that can help you and your fellow students. Some suggested keywords are: job searching, résumé writing, cover letters, interviewing skills, and professional image. Write down something new that you found to share.

_____
_____
_____
_____

THOUGHT TO PONDER

Learning isn't a means to an end; it is an end itself.

- Robert A. Heinlein

Here are some commonly asked interview questions. How would you answer them?

1. What are your strengths?_____
_____

2. What are your weaknesses? _____
_____

3. Why should we hire you?_____
_____

4. Where do you see yourself 5 years from now? _____
_____

5. Did you receive any scholarships and academic awards? _____
_____

6. How did you prepare for this interview? _____
_____

7. How do you plan to maintain your competency and remain current within your profession?_____
_____

8. How do you handle difficult people? _____
_____

9. What type of community and committee service have you performed? _____
_____

10. How do you feel about change?_____
_____

CHAPTER 11

Selected Topics

OBJECTIVES

Upon completion of this chapter, you should be able to:

Explain ethics and how they relate to health care professionals.

Discuss ethical issues that include confidentiality, respect, trust, death and dying, and euthanasia.

Discuss medical-legal issues that include malpractice, negligence, and the patient's rights.

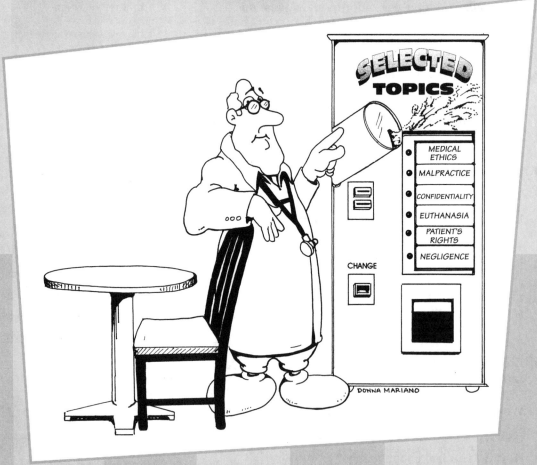

KEY TERMS

abandonment
advance directives
against medical advice
  (AMA)
battery
brain death
durable power of
  attorney
ethics

euthanasia
false imprisonment
fraud
Health Insurance
  Portability and
  Accountability Act
  (HIPAA)
hospice care
informed consent

invasion of privacy
malpractice
negligence
physical abuse
protocols
psychological abuse
scope of practice
sexual abuse
verbal abuse

INTRODUCTION

As a health care professional, you will be faced with ethical decisions almost daily. You will have access to confidential information concerning many aspects of a person's life. In addition, you are ethically bound to be current and competent with the level of care you will be administering to your patients. All health care professionals should familiarize themselves with and practice the stated code of ethics that their profession publishes. Health care professionals must also familiarize themselves with legal issues such as malpractice, negligence, and scope of practice.

MEDICAL ETHICS

Ethics is defined in dictionaries as moral principles or practices. In life, it means knowing the difference between right and wrong. In health care, it means conforming to accepted and professional standards of conduct. In both life and health care, ethical behavior is "doing the right thing in the right way." Ethics should govern and guide the way you act and the proper decisions you make. There are several situations in which ethics will influence decisions about patient care. These areas include confidentiality, respect, trust, and death and dying.

CONFIDENTIALITY

Confidentiality means keeping information private and not sharing it with inappropriate people. You will have access to information

217

concerning your patient that includes diagnosis, medical history, and lifestyle. You can discuss this information only with other health care professionals who are caring for this patient. You must use discretion when discussing patient information. Figure 11–1 shows some of the confidential information you may have access to in a medical chart.

For example, you may be in the cafeteria and say something as innocent such as, "I feel so bad for Mr. Smith in 408, his cancer biopsy was positive." Mr. Smith's family may be seated next to you and hear what you said. They may not know this information yet, and although you meant no harm, you have acted in an unprofessional and unethical manner.

One other aspect of confidentiality is that it is the physician's responsibility to tell the patient the results of tests or the diagnosis. You should discuss only the information related to the therapy or intervention you are performing.

What Do YOU Think?

Confidential Issues

What is wrong with the following situations?

1. You go home and tell one of your friends that you gave therapy to his or her cousin in the hospital today.
2. You tell someone at a party how surprised you were to find out that a patient you both know is an alcoholic.
3. You discuss a patient's past medical history or illness with another health care professional who is not involved in the case.
4. You tell a patient that he or she does not have the "bad" kind of cancer.

RESPECT

Each person deserves to be shown respect during the course of treatment. You may not agree with a patient's religious beliefs or choice of lifestyle, but again he or she may not agree with yours. Health care professionals are not to be judgmental. Your job is to deliver appropriate and considerate therapy to *all* your patients.

You will also encounter difficult patients who may be hostile, angry, or withdrawn. They may upset you with their actions, words, or refusal to comply with therapies. Again, you must respect their situation and place yourself in their shoes (or in this case hospital gown). They probably have good reason for their mood. You should remain calm and not argue with them. Arguing will only worsen the

MEDICAL HISTORY FORM

Date _____

Patient's name _____

Age	Date of birth	Sex	
Address	City	State	Zip code
Phone ( )			
Insurance company	Policy number		
Place of employment	Address		
Phone ( )	Job responsibilities		
Parent/Guardian if minor			
Address	City	State	Zip code
Phone ( )			

Family History:

List family members: (mother, father, brothers, sisters, grandparents, etc.)—ages and health status (if deceased write their age at the time of their death and the cause). List allergies and/or any conditions or diseases they may have or have had, such as asthma, arthritis, tuberculosis, diabetes, cancer, heart disease, hypertension, kidney disease, mental illness, depression, or any other health problems that you know of in your family.

_____

_____

_____

Patient's Past History: Mark the boxes to the right either "yes" or "no" for the following questions:*

Do you ever have or have you ever had any of the following: **(yes) (no)**

SKIN
Rashes, hives, itching or other skin irritations ( ) ( )

EYES, EARS, NOSE, THROAT
Headaches, dizziness, fainting ( ) ( )
Blurred or impaired vision ( ) ( )
Hearing loss or ringing in the ears ( ) ( )
Discharge from eyes or ears ( ) ( )
Sinus trouble/colds/allergies ( ) ( )
Asthma or hay fever ( ) ( )
Sore throats/hoarseness ( ) ( )

CARDIOPULMONARY
Shortness of breath ( ) ( )
Persistent cough or coughing up blood or other secretions ( ) ( )
Chills and/or fever ( ) ( )
Night sweats ( ) ( )
Tuberculosis or exposed to TB ( ) ( )

Scarlet fever or rheumatic fever ( ) ( )
Chest pain ( ) ( )
Heart palpitations or rapid heartbeat or pulse ( ) ( )
High blood pressure ( ) ( )
Swelling of hands and/or feet ( ) ( )

GASTROINTESTINAL
Heartburn or indigestion ( ) ( )
Nausea and/or vomiting ( ) ( )
Loss of appetite ( ) ( )
Belching or gas ( ) ( )
Peptic ulcer, gallbladder or liver disease ( ) ( )
Yellow jaundice or hepatitis ( ) ( )
Diarrhea or constipation ( ) ( )
Dysentery ( ) ( )
Rectal bleeding, hemorrhoids (piles) ( ) ( )
Tarry or clay-colored stools ( ) ( )

GLANDS
Weight gain or loss ( ) ( )

Diabetes ( ) ( )
Thyroid or goiter ( ) ( )
Swollen glands ( ) ( )

GENITOURINARY
Kidney disease or stones, or Bright's disease ( ) ( )
Painful, frequent or urgent urination ( ) ( )
Blood or pus in urine ( ) ( )
Sexually transmitted disease (venereal disease) ( ) ( )
Been sexually active with anyone who has AIDS or HIV or hepatitis ( ) ( )

NEUROMUSCULAR
Problems with becoming tired and/or upset easily ( ) ( )
Nervous breakdown/depression ( ) ( )
Poliomyelitis (infantile paralysis) ( ) ( )
Convulsions ( ) ( )
Joint and/or muscular pain ( ) ( )
Back pain or injury/osteomyelitis/rheumatism ( ) ( )

Are you currently taking any medications? **Yes** ( ) **No** ( )
If yes, please list them _____
Have you ever had or been treated for cancer or any tumors? ( ) ( )
Are you anemic or have you ever had to take iron medication? ( ) ( )
Do you use tobacco? ( ) ( )
What type? _____
Do you use IV drugs or alcohol? ( ) ( )

WOMEN ONLY
Painful menstrual periods ( ) ( )
Pregnancy/abortion/miscarriage ( ) ( )
Vaginal infection or discharge/abnormal bleeding ( ) ( )

Last menstrual period _____
Birth control _____
List dates of all operations/surgeries, injuries, and illnesses that required hospitalization:

_____

_____

Did you ever receive benefits from a medical insurance claim due to illness or injury? **Yes** ( ) **No** ( )
Were you ever rejected from the military or for employment? ( ) ( )
Were you absent from school/work in the past 10 years because of illness or injury? ( ) ( )
Did you ever file a Workers' Compensation claim? ( ) ( )
Did you ever seek psychological or psychiatric treatment? ( ) ( )

*Please use the back of this form to explain any "yes" answers. Thank you.

FIGURE 11-1

A sample of some of the confidential information to which you will have access situation. Calmness and consistent, considerate care will usually help the patient's outlook.

TRUST

Trust is an important ethical ingredient. A patient who trusts the health care professional will be more cooperative with the therapy and more forthcoming with information. Trust can be developed in several ways. First, you should be careful in handling the patient's personal belongings. You should follow your organization's policy and procedure in this matter. For example, most organizations require that a health care worker complete a checklist that lists the belongings of the patients while in the hospital.

Patients trust you to be dependable and have their therapy, bath, and food tray on time. This enhances trusting relationships. If a situation arises in which the schedule cannot be met, the circumstances should be explained to the patient.

Patients also trust that they will be safe and protected from harm. For example, patients often need transportation to other areas within the hospital. If certain rules are not followed, patient transport can be potentially dangerous. You need to make sure you know and follow your institution's safety guidelines for patient transport. For example, one common rule is to lock the wheels of transport devices such as gurneys (the moving beds) and wheelchairs when they are not moving. Can you imagine what would happen if an unattended patient in an unlocked wheelchair fell down a flight of steps?

Another way to protect the patient from harm is to report any suspected abuse. By law, health care workers must report any abuse of a person under 18 years of age. However, you should report all cases regardless of age to the proper person. In many cases, the proper person is the nurse in charge of that area or the social service department.

Abuse can take on four specific forms. **Physical abuse** results from actual contact, usually resulting in a visible injury. Although physical abuse can sometimes be evident by bruise marks on the patient, neglect such as not feeding or providing a safe environment can also be classified as physical abuse.

Verbal abuse occurs when spoken words are meant to hurt another person's self-esteem. This can make a person feel unimportant, worthless, or bad about themselves.

Psychological abuse is sometimes harder to see or hear. This abuse results in a fearful state for the person being abused. This can take the form of vicious threats such as, "If you wet the bed one more time, I'll let you sleep in it."

Sexual abuse is any inappropriate sexual touch or act. As a health care practitioner, you will be in a position of authority over patients. This authority comes from your expert knowledge. The practitioner-patient relationship gives you control over many situations. Add to this the fact that patients are often in very vulnerable states and you could have the potential for sexual abuse. Therefore, sexual relations with patients is unethical and would interfere with the therapeutic relationship that should exist between a practitioner and patient.

Whatever houses I may visit, I will come for the benefit of the sick, remaining free of all intentional injustice, of all mischief and in particular of sexual relationships with both male and female persons.
- Hippocratic Oath

What Do YOU Think?

Sources of Abuse

Abuse can come from family members, friends, or complete strangers. However, abuse can also be caused by health care workers. Can you think of examples of when health care workers could abuse their patients? What would you do if you witnessed abuse?

DEATH AND DYING

Death and dying is an ethical issue we must all face. As health care professionals, we will deal with this issue on a more frequent basis. Not only may we witness death occur during a cardiac or respiratory arrest, but we will also experience the process of dying through our terminally ill patients. Therefore, it is important to examine many of your own feelings and beliefs concerning death and dying. The first step is to understand what usually occurs during the process of dying. Dr. Elizabeth Kübler-Ross did a great deal of work with patients dying of terminal illness. Her extensive study led to the identification of the following five stages of grieving that occurs during the dying process:

• Denial

• Anger

• Bargaining

• Depression

• Acceptance

Denial, usually the first stage of the grieving process, occurs after the patient is made aware of the terminal diagnosis. Here, the patient denies having the disease with statements such as, "The tests must be wrong" or "It can't be that bad."

The second stage, anger, usually follows denial, and the patient becomes hostile and bitter about the situation. The health care worker may become the target of the patient's anger. Remember, do not take any anger directed at you personally. It is best to be supportive and understanding with the patient at all times.

The third stage identified is bargaining. During this stage, the patient bargains according to his or her spiritual beliefs. The patient may plead, "Please let me live to see my grandchild." Again, your best response is to actively listen and provide support.

Depression represents the fourth stage of the grieving process. This is usually when the patient becomes withdrawn and extremely sad. The patient may break down and cry. Again, your support is what is needed. You may even find yourself getting emotional with the patient, and a gentle touch at the appropriate time may help.

The fifth and final stage is acceptance. At this time, the patient will want to complete unfinished business, and your support in facilitating this is important. A certain calm may be experienced by the patient during this stage.

Patients may move through these stages in different orders; however, you can usually identify what stage they are in by their moods, actions, and language used (see Figure 11–2). Understanding the stages will also help you cope with their death. For example, you may have a patient you have come to know very well over time. After being diagnosed as having a terminal disease, the patient may become angry or withdraw from you. It is important that you understand that this as a normal part of the grieving process and not personally directed at you.

A special part of the health care system has been developed to care for terminally ill patients; it is called **hospice care**. Hospice care helps the patient and family throughout the grieving process and allows the patient to die with dignity, usually at home where the patient feels most comfortable.

DENIAL	"I'm too young to die." "The tests must be wrong." "You've made a mistake."
ANGER	"Get out of my room!" "This hospital is worthless!" "I hate my treatments!"
BARGAINING	"Please let me live to see my grandson graduate." "If you let me live, I'll promise to . . ."
DEPRESSION	"Leave me alone." "I don't want any more treatments."
ACCEPTANCE	"I have so much to tell people." "I need to get my affairs in order."

FIGURE 11-2
Verbal examples of the stages of death and dying

EUTHANASIA

The right to die is a controversial issue. **Euthanasia** technically means an "easy death." In health care, it is the concept of medically assisting another to die. Euthanasia can be divided into a passive or active form. Passive euthanasia is the process of withholding treatment that could sustain a life. Active euthanasia is actively assisting the patient in dying.

What Do YOU Think?

Mercy Killing

Active voluntary euthanasia can be termed mercy killing. What are your thoughts concerning this concept? Can you find any recent news articles related to this concept?

The question arises whether advanced life support should be withheld or withdrawn from certain terminally ill patients. Although death is a natural progression of life, there are still many questions about just what death is. **Brain death** is defined as the irreversible cessation of all functions of the brain. This state goes beyond a comatose (coma) state in which the brain is still functioning to maintain life and the patient still has the ability for conscious thought.

With advances in technology, life support equipment can maintain someone's life who is brain dead for months and even years. This state of being is called a persistent vegetative state; the patient is in a permanent state of unconsciousness, and the vital functions of the body are performed by machines.

Many would argue that someone in a vegetative state is really not alive. This raises the question of one's quality of life. The quality of life looks at the individual's potential ability to return to a conscious state and function at a level that maintains qualities such as awareness and human interaction. People who believe in the quality of life issues believe the major goal of health care should be to maintain the quality of life of the individual.

What Do YOU Think?

Above and Beyond the Call?

Depending on the physician's beliefs, treatments can take various forms. For example, physicians who believe all measures should be taken at all times to continue life will use extraordinary means. Extraordinary means include using all medicines, treatments, and operations, regardless of expense, pain, or other inconveniences to patient or family. What do you think about extraordinary care? Should expense be a consideration?

LEARNER:

Go to page 237 and complete the Critical Thinking and Application Activities 11–1, 11–2, and 11–3.

LEGAL ISSUES

The patient's well-being is entrusted to the various health care practitioners providing care. Each state has written laws or statutes that define what certified or licensed health care workers can do. This is called the **scope of practice**. You cannot exceed your scope of practice because this is what you were specifically trained to do and legally allowed to do. State boards regulate the licensee or certificate holder and can revoke the license for violation of scope of practice or involvement in other stated offenses such as drug abuse, sexual abuse, felonies, and so on.

In addition to a defined scope of practice, each health care organization has its own guidelines and established ways of doing things. These guidelines can take the form of policies, procedures, and protocols. **Protocols** help standardize care and help establish "how and when to do your specific procedures and interventions" in specific situations. For example, a patient safety protocol may state that all side rails must be raised when transporting a patient on a gurney.

NEGLIGENCE AND MALPRACTICE

Two general types of legal actions can be taken against a health care worker in the line of duty: **negligence** and **malpractice**. Negligence is the failure to give reasonable care and can be intentional or unintentional. Intentional negligence includes battery, false imprisonment, abandonment, invasion of privacy, and fraud.

Battery means using touch or force without the patient's consent. This includes doing a procedure without having the patient's proper consent. Each patient has the right to determine what can and cannot be done. All health care facilities should have a consent form that the patient must sign before admission and certain procedures. Any type of surgical procedure requires an **informed consent**. Informed means that the patient has been instructed about what the procedure entails. All consents require a witness 21 years of age or older and should be signed in black ink. Consents can be given over the telephone in certain situations. Accepting telephone consent requires two people to listen at the same time.

False imprisonment is restraining a person against his or her will. Sometimes it may be necessary to use restraining measures to prevent patients from doing harm to themselves or others. However, one should not restrain a patient because he or she is being difficult or because it would make the health care worker's job easier. In health care, a physician order is required to restrain any patient. Some patients may insist on leaving the health care institution, even when it may not be in their best interest. If a patient insists on leaving, he or she may be signed out **"against medical advice" (AMA)**, meaning that a health care worker has advised the patient against leaving and has explained the possible dangers of disrupting treatment.

Abandonment is leaving a patient who needs additional care. For example, you notice a patient is drowning in his or her own secretions and you simply leave the room instead of clearing the secretions. This is a form of abandonment.

Invasion of privacy is any public discussion of private information concerning your patient. This includes discussing a diagnosis, biographical information, and lifestyle preferences. Because you have access to privileged information, you must always maintain confidentiality. Follow the rule to discuss patient issues only with other health care professionals, and then only when that discussion adds to the treatment of the patient.

> **W**hat I may see or hear in the course of treatment or even outside of treatment in regard to the life of men, which on no account must be noised abroad, I will keep to myself holding such things shameful to be spoken about.
>
> - Hippocratic Oath

Invasion of privacy also includes the patient's body being handled by someone not involved in care or the patient's personal belongings being handled without permission. Protect your patients' privacy by knocking before entering a room, drawing curtains while performing procedures, and protecting them from exposure from hospital gowns. In addition, allow visitors time alone with the patient, and do not listen to conversations and telephone calls.

Privacy is such an important issue that federal legislation was enacted to further protect the confidentiality of medical records and information. The **Health Insurance Portability and Accountability Act (HIPAA)** of 1996 established a well-defined set of regulations concerning protection of patient privacy. This federal legislation covered the following three areas:

1. Insurance Portability: Ensures individuals' ability to maintain health insurance coverage when they switch from one health plan to another. In addition, it prevents health plans from denying coverage due to a preexisting condition.

2. Administrative Simplification: This part of the act requires health care providers and health insurance plans to standardize the process they use to exchange electronic information and implement policies to protect this exchange of information as it relates to patient confidentiality.

3. Privacy and Security: This section of the act requires that health care providers use methods to ensure that a patient's medical information is secure and private.

All health care organizations should have HIPAA policies and training sessions that demonstrate compliance with this important federal legislation. Information about an individual and their health information are considered Protected Health Information (PHI) and include the following:

- Name
- Medical record number
- Social Security number
- Address
- Date of birth
- Diagnosis
- Medical history
- Medications

Some highlights of policies common to many organizations as a result of HIPAA are:

- Patients must sign a release before any PHI information can be released.
- Patients should be made aware of HIPAA, how their information is protected, and whom to contact if they suspect a violation.
- Patients have a right to access and view their health information in most cases.
- Patients can request to amend or correct their PHI if they feel it is in error.
- PHI should only be available to staff on a "need to know in order to do their job" basis.
- Oral communication is a common breach of confidentiality, and policies should address this also.
- Medical information should be physically (locked) and electronically secured (codes and passwords) to prevent unauthorized access.
- Be careful of photocopies and faxed information others can view.
- Medical information should be properly disposed.

Making sure everyone in your facility is HIPAA compliant not only protects the patients but also the employees and the financial situation of the organization. Violations of the HIPAA act can result in penalties and fines up to $250,000 and 10 years imprisonment.

Fraud consists of the intentional withholding or modification of information. For example, modifying a chart to cover up a medication error is a fraudulent act. Negligence can also be unintentional, such as forgetting to put the side rails up or not immediately cleaning up a spill.

The medical term *mal* means bad. Therefore, malpractice can be thought of as bad practice. Malpractice is any professional misconduct or lack of competency that results in injury to the patient. Performing a procedure incorrectly or practicing outside your scope of practice or competency level constitutes malpractice.

TEST Yourself

Negligence or Malpractice

Negligence and malpractice are often confused. Identify each of the following as an act of negligence or malpractice.

1. Applying a heat pack that burns a patient
2. Performing a procedure that is outside your scope of practice
3. Restraining a patient because you are tired of him pulling out the intravenous line
4. Performing cardiopulmonary resuscitation (CPR) incorrectly

THE PATIENT CARE PARTNERSHIP

When a patient requires health care, the quality of that care is enhanced with a true partnership between the patient and the health care institution. The American Hospital Association has developed the Patient Care Partnership document, which assists all parties (patient, family members, and the health care institution) in defining and understanding their expectations, rights, and responsibilities (Figure 11-3).

Patients and their family members should be aware of their basic rights, often referred to as the Patient Care Partnership.

A brief summary of these basic rights include the right to:

- Considerate and respectful care
- Be told about the care that they will receive
- Examine the costs of their care
- Have their privacy protected
- Be involved in decisions concerning their care
- Be able to accept or refuse any treatment or procedure
- Be told of hospital rules and regulations

The Patient Care Partnership:
Understanding Expectations, Rights and Responsibilities

When you need hospital care, your doctor and the nurses and other professionals at our hospital are committed to working with you and your family to meet your health care needs. Our dedicated doctors and staff serve the community in all its ethnic, religious and economic diversity. Our goal is for you and your family to have the same care and attention we would want for our families and ourselves.

The sections explain some of the basics about how you can expect to be treated during your hospital stay. They also cover what we will need from you to care for you better. If you have questions at any time, please ask them. Unasked or unanswered questions can add to the stress of being in the hospital. Your comfort and confidence in your care are very important to us.

What to Expect During Your Hospital Stay

- **High quality hospital care.** Our first priority is to provide you the care you need, when you need it, with skill, compassion, and respect. Tell your caregivers if you have concerns about your care or if you have pain. You have the right to know the identity of doctors, nurses and others involved in your care, and you have the right to know when they are students, residents or other trainees.

- **A clean and safe environment.** Our hospital works hard to keep you safe. We use special policies and procedures to avoid mistakes in your care and keep you free from abuse or neglect. If anything unexpected and significant happens during your hospital stay, you will be told what happened, and any resulting changes in your care will be discussed with you.

- **Involvement in your care.** You and your doctor often make decisions about your care before you go to the hospital. Other times, especially in emergencies, those decisions are made during your hospital stay. When decision-making takes place, it should include:

  ➤ *Discussing your medical condition and information about medically appropriate treatment choices.* To make informed decisions with your doctor, you need to understand:
    - The benefits and risks of each treatment.
    - Whether your treatment is experimental or part of a research study.
    - What you can reasonably expect from your treatment and any long-term effects it might have on your quality of life.
    - What you and your family will need to do after you leave the hospital.
    - The financial consequences of using uncovered services or out-of-network providers.
    Please tell your caregivers if you need more information about treatment choices.

  ➤ *Discussing your treatment plan.* When you enter the hospital, you sign a general consent to treatment. In some cases, such as surgery or experimental treatment, you may be asked to confirm in writing that you understand what is planned and agree to it. This process protects your right to consent to or refuse a treatment. Your doctor will explain the medical consequences of refusing recommended treatment. It also protects your right to decide if you want to participate in a research study.

(Continues)

FIGURE 11-3
The Patient Care Partnership (Reprinted with permission of the American Hospital Association, copyright 2003)

➤ *Getting information from you.* Your caregivers need complete and correct information about your health and coverage so that they can make good decisions about your care. That includes:
 – Past illnesses, surgeries or hospital stays.
 – Past allergic reactions.
 – Any medicines or dietary supplements (such as vitamins and herbs) that you are taking.
 – Any network or admission requirements under your health plan.

➤ *Understanding your health care goals and values.* You may have health care goals and values or spiritual beliefs that are important to your well-being. They will be taken into account as much as possible throughout your hospital stay. Make sure your doctor, your family and your care team know your wishes.

➤ *Understanding who should make decisions when you cannot.* If you have signed a health care power of attorney stating who should speak for you if you become unable to make health care decisions for yourself, or a "living will" or "advance directive" that states your wishes about end-of-life care; give copies to your doctor, your family and your care team. If you or your family need help making difficult decisions, counselors, chaplains and others are available to help.

• **Protection of your privacy.** We respect the confidentiality of your relationship with your doctor and other caregivers, and the sensitive information about your health and health care that are part of that relationship. State and federal laws and hospital operating policies protect the privacy of your medical information. You will receive a Notice of Privacy Practices that describes the ways that we use, disclose and safeguard patient information and that explains how you can obtain a copy of information from our records about your care.

• **Preparing you and your family for when you leave the hospital.** Your doctor works with hospital staff and professionals in your community. You and your family also play an important role in your care. The success of your treatment often depends on your efforts to follow medication, diet and therapy plans. Your family may need to help care for you at home.

You can expect us to help you identify sources of follow-up care and to let you know if our hospital has a financial interest in any referrals. As long as you agree that we can share information about your care with them, we will coordinate our activities with your caregivers outside the hospital. You can also expect to receive information and, where possible, training about the self-care you will need when you go home.

• **Help with your bill and filing insurance claims.** Our staff will file claims for you with health care insurers or other programs such as Medicare and Medicaid. They also will help your doctor with needed documentation. Hospital bills and insurance coverage are often confusing. If you have questions about your bill, contact our business office. If you need help understanding your insurance coverage or health plan, start with your insurance company or health benefits manager. If you do not have health coverage, we will try to help you and your family find financial help or make other arrangements. We need your help with collecting needed information and other requirements to obtain coverage or assistance.

While you are here, you will receive more detailed notices about some of the rights you have as a hospital patient and how to exercise them. We are always interested in improving. If you have questions, comments, or concerns, please contact _____.

FIGURE 11-3
(Continued)

Although many may think of health care as confined to the hospital, this is far from accurate. With the many recent changes in health care in the United States, more and more care is occurring in outpatient clinics, rehabilitation centers, physicians' offices, and long-term care facilities. Long-term care facility residents have an additional set of rights that are guaranteed to them. These rights are listed in a document called the Resident's Bill of Rights, and include the following:

- Residents can freely choose their physician, treatment, and care, and decide whether they will participate in any research project.
- Residents are protected from any type of abuse or chemical and physical restraints. Chemical restraints include sedatives to "control" the patient and make it easier to care for them.
- Residents should have a choice in their activities and schedules.
- Residents can voice criticism or complaints without any fear of retaliation.
- Residents can organize in groups for purposes of religious or social activities.
- Residents have access to information on their medical benefits and records. In addition, they can look at evaluation results of the long-term facility, including any identified deficiencies.
- Residents can manage their own moneys and possessions.
- Residents have unlimited access to their immediate family and relatives. If a married couple is staying at the facility, they have the right to share a room.

RIGHT TO DIE ISSUES

Modern medicine may have the ability to prolong a life with advanced technology, but some patients choose to die naturally. Patients with no hope of recovery can request that no extra measures be given to resuscitate them.

Patients may have an **advance directive** signed. This is often called a living will because it states the patient's wishes concerning the handling of his or her body while still living. For example, it specifies what can and cannot be done to sustain life if the patient cannot make that decision. This can occur with a patient who is unconscious and in a vegetative state or someone who has just stopped breathing. Figure 11–4 is an example of a living will.

Patients can also give others the ability to make decisions for them if they are unable to. This is a called a health care proxy, which is a legal document that identifies someone else to make the decisions for them. A legal document that identifies another individual to make decisions for the patient if they are unable to is called **durable power of attorney**. Figure 11–5 is an example of a living will with a health care proxy included.

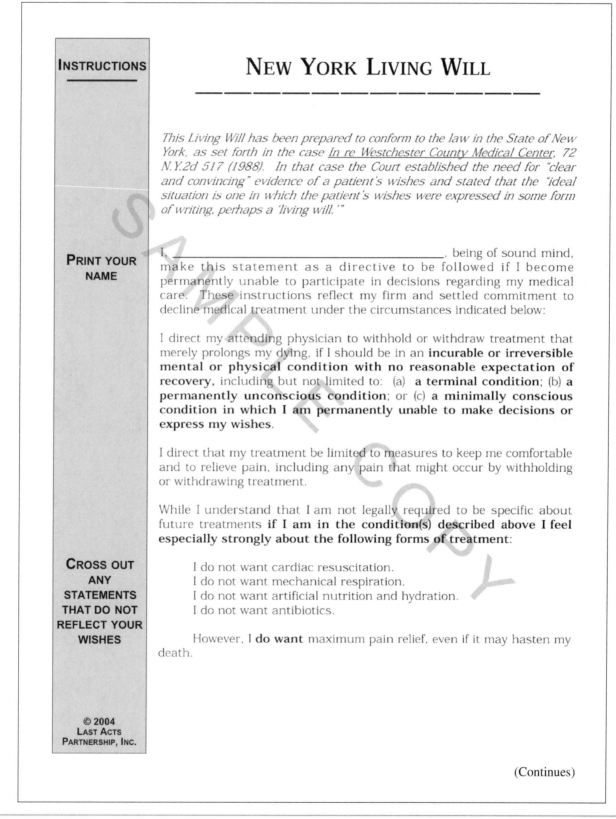

NEW YORK LIVING WILL

— — — — — — — — — — — — — — —

INSTRUCTIONS

This Living Will has been prepared to conform to the law in the State of New York, as set forth in the case <u>In re Westchester County Medical Center</u>, 72 N.Y.2d 517 (1988). In that case the Court established the need for "clear and convincing" evidence of a patient's wishes and stated that the "ideal situation is one in which the patient's wishes were expressed in some form of writing, perhaps a 'living will.'"

PRINT YOUR NAME

I, _____, being of sound mind, make this statement as a directive to be followed if I become permanently unable to participate in decisions regarding my medical care. These instructions reflect my firm and settled commitment to decline medical treatment under the circumstances indicated below:

I direct my attending physician to withhold or withdraw treatment that merely prolongs my dying, if I should be in an **incurable or irreversible mental or physical condition with no reasonable expectation of recovery,** including but not limited to: (a) **a terminal condition;** (b) **a permanently unconscious condition;** or (c) **a minimally conscious condition in which I am permanently unable to make decisions or express my wishes.**

I direct that my treatment be limited to measures to keep me comfortable and to relieve pain, including any pain that might occur by withholding or withdrawing treatment.

While I understand that I am not legally required to be specific about future treatments **if I am in the condition(s) described above I feel especially strongly about the following forms of treatment:**

CROSS OUT ANY STATEMENTS THAT DO NOT REFLECT YOUR WISHES

    I do not want cardiac resuscitation.
    I do not want mechanical respiration.
    I do not want artificial nutrition and hydration.
    I do not want antibiotics.

    However, I **do want** maximum pain relief, even if it may hasten my death.

(Continues)

FIGURE 11-4
Sample living will form (copyright 2004 Last Acts Partnership, Inc. All rights reserved.)

	NEW YORK LIVING WILL — PAGE 2 OF 2
ADD PERSONAL INSTRUCTIONS (IF ANY)	Other directions:
	These directions express my legal right to refuse treatment, under the law of New York. I intend my instructions to be carried out, unless I have rescinded them in a new writing or by clearly indicating that I have changed my mind.
SIGN AND DATE THE DOCUMENT AND PRINT YOUR ADDRESS	Signed _____ Date _____ Address _____
WITNESSING PROCEDURE	I declare that the person who signed this document appeared to execute the living will willingly and free from duress. He or she signed (or asked another to sign for him or her) this document in my presence.
YOUR WITNESSES MUST SIGN AND PRINT THEIR ADDRESSES	Witness 1 _____ Address _____ Witness 2 _____ Address _____
© 2004 LAST ACTS PARTNERSHIP, INC.	*Courtesy of* Last Acts Partnership, Inc.　　12/00 1620 Eye Street, NW, Suite 200 . Washington, DC 20006 800-989-9455

FIGURE 11-4
(Continued)

NEW YORK
HEALTHCARE PROXY

_____

(1) I, _____, hereby appoint:

(name)

_____

(name, home address and telephone number of agent)

_____

as my healthcare agent to make any and all healthcare decisions for me, except to the extent that I state otherwise. My agent does know my wishes regarding artificial nutrition and hydration.

This Healthcare Proxy shall take effect in the event I become unable to make my own healthcare decisions.

(2) Optional instructions: I direct my agent to make healthcare decisions in accord with my wishes and limitations as stated below, or as he or she otherwise knows.

(3) Name of substitute or fill-in agent if the person I appoint above is unable, unwilling or unavailable to act as my healthcare agent.

_____

(name, home address and telephone number of alternate agent)

_____

(4) Donation of Organs at Death: Upon my death:

[ ] I **do not** wish to donate my organs, tissues or parts.
[ ] I **do** wish to be an organ donor and upon my death I wish to donate:

(Continued)

INSTRUCTIONS
_____

PRINT YOUR NAME

PRINT NAME, HOME ADDRESS AND TELEPHONE NUMBER OF YOUR AGENT

ADD PERSONAL INSTRUCTIONS (IF ANY)

PRINT NAME, HOME ADDRESS AND TELEPHONE NUMBER OF YOUR ALTERNATE AGENT

ORGAN DONATION (OPTIONAL)

© 2004 LAST ACTS PARTNERSHIP, INC.

FIGURE 11-5
A health care proxy (copyright 2004 Last Acts Partnership, Inc. All rights reserved.)

	NEW YORK HEALTHCARE PROXY — PAGE 2 OF 2

ORGAN DONATION (OPTIONAL) CONTINUED	[ ] (a) Any needed organs, tissues, or parts;
	OR
	[ ] (b) The following organs, tissues, or parts
	_____
	_____
	
	[ ] (c) My gift is for the following purposes:
	    (put a line through any of the following you do not want)
	      (i) Transplant
	      (ii) Therapy
	      (iii) Research
	      (iv) Education

ENTER A DURATION OR A CONDITION (IF ANY)	(5) Unless I revoke it, this proxy shall remain in effect indefinitely, or until the date or condition I have stated below. This proxy shall expire (specific date or conditions, if desired): _____ _____
SIGN AND DATE THE DOCUMENT AND PRINT YOUR ADDRESS	(6) Signature _____ Date _____ Address _____
WITNESSING PROCEDURE	**Statement by Witnesses** (must be 18 or older) I declare that the person who signed this document appeared to execute the proxy willingly and free from duress. He or she signed (or asked another to sign for him or her) this document in my presence. I am not the person appointed as proxy by this document.
YOUR WITNESSES MUST SIGN AND PRINT THEIR ADDRESSES	Witness 1 _____ Address_____ Witness 2 _____ Address _____
© 2004 LAST ACTS PARTNERSHIP, INC.	*Courtesy of* **Last Acts Partnership, Inc.** 12/00 1620 Eye Street, NW, Suite 200 Washington, DC 20006 800-989-9455

FIGURE 11-5
(Continued)

Living wills often result in a notation in the chart or a physician order specifying the patient's wishes. For example, the physician may write an order in the chart that states "do not resuscitate" (DNR). It is important to know whether your patient has this order in the event that he or she ceases to breathe or the heart stops during your treatment or interaction.

SUMMARY

Medical ethics must be considered by all current and future health care professionals. Confidentiality, respect, and trust coupled with safe and appropriate care will serve as guidelines for ethical treatment of patients. In addition, you and your patients will be faced with issues such as death and dying, euthanasia, and other issues that will cause examination of your personal beliefs.

Legal issues are also an important consideration for all health care practitioners. It is important to understand your particular scope of practice so that you understand what it is you can and cannot do. You must also understand the terms *negligence* and *malpractice* and prevent their occurrences in the practice of your chosen profession.

A summary of standards that will protect you and the patient follows:

1. Know your scope of practice and keep within it.

2. Remain current with your knowledge and use only approved, correct procedures.

3. Know and follow your institution's policies and procedures concerning informed consent.

4. Know your institution's safety policies and procedures. Especially important are fire safety, patient transportation, and handling of accidents, hazardous materials, and defective equipment.

5. Keep all information confidential and give considerate care to all patients.

6. Maintain a professional image in dress and attitude.

7. Make sure the procedure is to be performed on that particular patient. This includes verification of the physician order and checking the patient's wrist name band (Figure 11–6).

8. Report any errors or accidents immediately, and document them with an incident report.

9. Do not accept money or tips for any services. However, taking a piece of chocolate cake (my favorite) offered in a patient's home may be acceptable, depending on the circumstances.

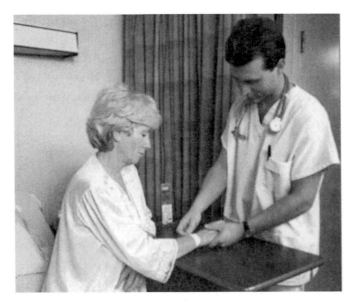

FIGURE 11-6
Always check the wrist
name tag to ensure that the
proper patient is receiving
care.

LEARNER:

Go to page 238 and complete the Critical Thinking and
Application Activities 11–4, 11–5, 11–6, 11–7, and 11–8.

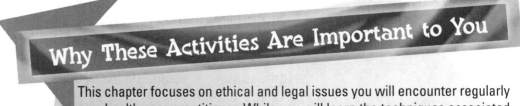

Why These Activities Are Important to You

This chapter focuses on ethical and legal issues you will encounter regularly
as a health care practitioner. While you will learn the techniques associated
with the practice of your chosen profession, the ethical and legal issues are
less visible and easy to demonstrate. These issues require thought and reflection. Anyone choosing a health care profession should give careful consideration to these issues.

CRITICAL THINKING AND APPLICATION ACTIVITIES

11-1   Ethical and Unethical Situations

Give an example of an ethical and unethical situation for each of the categories.

1. Confidentiality

    Ethical situation: _____

    _____

    _____

    Unethical situation: _____

    _____

    _____

2. Respect

    Ethical situation: _____

    _____

    _____

    Unethical situation: _____

    _____

    _____

3. Trust

    Ethical situation: _____

    _____

    _____

    Unethical situation: _____

    _____

    _____

11-2   Ethical Issues

Research the following topics:

- Death and dying
- Euthanasia
- Hospice care

You can use the Internet or library, or you can call a local hospice unit. In one paragraph, write the most interesting fact you learned about these topics that was not included in this chapter, and share it with the class.

1. Death and dying: _____

_____

_____

_____

2. Euthanasia: _____

_____

_____

_____

3. Hospice care: _____

_____

_____

_____

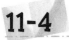 **11-3 Ethical Debates**

Pair off in groups of four to six. Choose an ethical topic to debate. For example, is physician-assisted death justifiable? If so, under what circumstances? Your group should develop an ethical dilemma or question and then debate the issue and list the various viewpoints. Remember, there are no clear right or wrong answers, and you should listen to the differing viewpoints of others with respect.

Your group ethical dilemma or question: _____

_____

_____

_____

Various viewpoints: _____

_____

_____

_____

_____

_____

11-4 Getting to Know Your Profession

Research two health care professions that interest you. Call or write their national or local offices and obtain their scope of practice and code of ethics. In addition, obtain the information needed to contact the malpractice insurance carrier for that profession. (You will need this for the next activity.)

Scope of practice: _____

_____

_____

Code of ethics:_____

_____

_____

11-5   Malpractice Insurance

Contact the insurance carrier from the information you received in the previous activity and request a student malpractice policy and application be sent to you. Highlight the important points and coverage of that policy below and share with your class.

_____

_____

_____

_____

_____

11-6   Safety Poster Presentation

Safety Issues

As health care professionals, we must concern ourselves not only with our safety but also with that of the patients. The health care institution is legally bound to provide a safe environment for its employees, patients, and visitors.

Safety issues lend themselves well to poster presentations, which can highlight and emphasize the most important points. A poster presentation should minimally include the following:

- A title
- Brief text boxes that explain the major points or issues
- Bulleted lists, if they help highlight information
- Pictures, diagrams, or illustrations to give a visual representation

This activity will allow you to explore safety issues that will affect you and/or your patient. Choose one of the topics listed below, make a poster presentation, and share it with your class.

- Proper body mechanics when lifting
- Patient transportation
- Fire safety
- Accident prevention
- Electrical safety
- Handling of hazardous wastes
- Accidental needle stick prevention
- Universal precautions

11-7   Case Study

You are working in an outpatient surgery clinic. In the hallway you hear two of your coworkers discussing the cosmetic surgery that one of the patients is receiving. This is not a medical discussion and is more of a gossip session with derogatory comments concerning the patient's vanity. They are speaking loudly enough that you feel people in the visitors' waiting area can hear their conversation. What should you do in this situation?

_____

_____

_____

_____

_____

11-8   Internet Activity

Using Internet search engines, find additional material on selected topics that can help you and your fellow students. Some suggested keywords are: medical ethics, HIPAA regulations, euthanasia, malpractice, and hospice. Write down something new that you found to share.

_____

_____

_____

_____

THOUGHTS TO PONDER

When does life begin?

When does life end?

How would you define quality of life?

Is assisted death justified?

Should organs of a brain-dead person be harvested and used to save other lives?

GLOSSARY

abandonment: leaving a patient who needs additional care

acronym: a word made from the first letter of other words

active listening: when the mind is focusing on both the message and the speaker during the communication process

advance directives: document stating the patient's wishes concerning the handling of his or her body while the person is still living

against medical advice (AMA): when a patient insists on leaving the health care institution and has been advised against leaving and told of the dangers of disrupting treatment

analogy: forces cross-connections between two unlike things

bad stress: when anxiety reaches a level that interferes with performance or stops performance entirely

battery: the use of touch or force without the patient's consent

brainstorming: when a group of people get together and come up with ideas concerning an opportunity or issue

brain death: irreversible cessation of all functions of the brain

caring attitude: sincerity, empathy, respect, and consideration toward others

charting: the process of recording information on a patient's chart; the chart is a legal document that includes confidential material on patient history, current medical status, and recovery process

chief complaint: the patient's reason for seeking medical help

classical conditioning: repeated actions that lead to a desired behavior

closed-ended questions: questions that can be answered with a simple yes or no response

cognitive processes: the complex mental activities that constitute thinking

cohesiveness: the degree to which members work together

communication: the exchange of messages, information, thoughts, ideas, and feelings

communication process: the process of communicating, which includes a sender presenting a clear message to a receiver who relays feedback

competency: being capable of doing something well

complacency: an interference during the communication process that results in the message getting through but its being acted on only half-heartedly or not at all

conformity: changing one's opinion or behavior in response to pressure from a group

constructive concern: converting useless worries into positive improvements

cover letter: accompanies a résumé and helps demonstrate interest in the job that is being sought by getting the attention of the employer

creative thinking: the generation of ideas that results in the improvement of the efficiency or the effectiveness of the system

critical thinking: the ability to gather and analyze information to solve problems or create new opportunities

customer relations: refers to the way clients (patients and visitors) are treated by the employees of a business

decision making: the act of making an informed choice between a number of alternatives in order to solve a problem and/or maximize an opportunity

decoding: translating a message into a perception

deductive reasoning: a form of logical thinking in which a true conclusion is based on true facts called premises

depression: remaining sad for prolonged periods, which interferes with the ability to perform daily activities

diagonal communication: the flow of communication between departments or people that are on different lateral planes of the organizational chart

directed thinking: a conscious effort made to solve a specific problem or situation through learning, reasoning, and decision making

downward communication: formal flow of communication from people with formal power to staff employees

durable power of attorney: a legal document that identifies another individual to make decisions for the patient if the patient is unable to

empathy: the ability to feel and understand what others are going through

encoding: the process of converting ideas or messages into words, diagrams, graphs, or reports

endorphins: the body's natural painkillers

enunciation: the clarity with which words are pronounced

environmental communication barriers: when the environment interferes with the communication process

ethics: conforming to accepted and professional standards of conduct

euthanasia: medically assisting another to die

false imprisonment: restraining a person against his or her will

formal communication channels: communication flow that can be seen by viewing an organizational chart or flowchart that is established by the way the organization is put together

formal group: a collection of people who share clear goals and expectations along with established rules of conduct

fraud: consists of the intentional withholding or modification of information

functional résumé: a list of one's experiences in terms of skills previously used on jobs or throughout one's educational career

goals: specific accomplishments which one aims to achieve

good stress: helps motivate a person to be up for a task

gossip: mostly based on rumors and becomes more personal in nature; is usually directed at an individual or group of individuals

group dynamics: the study of how people interact in groups

groupthink: the unquestioning acceptance of the group's beliefs and behaviors

Health Insurance Portability and Accountability Act (HIPAA): Federal legislation enacted in 1996 that established a well-defined set of regulations concerning protection of patient privacy

hearing: the process, function, or power of perceiving sound; requires concentration while blocking out external and internal distractions

horizontal communication: when departments or groups of people on the same level of the organizational chart talk with each other

hospice care: a special part of the health care system that helps patients and their families throughout the grieving process and allows the patient to die with dignity, usually at home, where the patient feels most comfortable

inductive reasoning: making the best guess based on premises or facts

informal communication channels: communication that is established through the "grapevine"

informal groups: a loose association of people without stated rules or goals

informed consent: any type of surgical procedure requires that a patient sign a consent form stating that he or she has been instructed about what the procedure entails

interview: an evaluation of a potential employee's job skills, knowledge, character, and oral communication skills

intimate space: the distance of 0 to 18 inches away from a patient

invasion of privacy: any public discussion of private information concerning your patient

lateral thinking: a creative type of thinking that generates new ideas by connecting previously unrelated concepts

lateral communication: communication at the same level of the organizational chart

leadership: a set of behaviors, attitudes, and values that enables the leader to motivate and direct others to act

listening: paying attention and focusing on the sounds that are heard

logical thinking: the ability to reason both deductively and inductively in a given situation

long-range goals: goals to be accomplished within the next few years

malpractice: any professional misconduct or lack of competency that results in injury to the patient

meditation: focusing your attention while at the same time clearing your mind of thought

medium-range goals: goals to be accomplished within the next 6 months to 1 year

mnemonics: words, rhymes, or formulas that aid your memory

negative attitude: maintaining a pessimistic outlook during situations

negligence: the failure to give reasonable care; can be intentional or unintentional

nonverbal communication: the use of behavior such as facial expressions, gestures, body language, and touch to communicate

norms: rules within particular groups that people in particular roles are expected to adhere to

objective: the end task that is to be accomplished

open-ended questions: questions that require an explanation as a response

oral communication: a form of verbal communication in which words are exchanged either face-to-face or through another means, such as a telephone

organizational chart: a chart that shows the flow of communication, the relationships of various departments, and the lines of authority within an organization

personal communication barriers: when a problem exists within an individual or the person with whom the communication is taking place that interferes with the communication process

personal space: the distance of approximately 18 inches to 4 feet away from a patient

physical abuse: results from actual contact, usually resulting in a visible injury

plateau period: period when little or no progress is made toward desired goals

positive attitude: maintaining a optimistic outlook during situations

procrastination: putting things off until the last minute

profession: an area of specialization

professional image: enhancing and demonstrating one's professionalism; for example, by becoming actively involved in a professional organization

pronunciation: the correctness with which words are pronounced

protocols: guidelines and established ways of doing things within each health care organization

psychological abuse: results in a fearful state for the person being abused; can be in the form of vicious threats

punctuality: being on time

reframing: changing the perception on a situation

respect: valuing patients and coworkers by being courteous and understanding even in the most difficult situations

résumé: a short summary about oneself that informs potential employees about education, experience, and qualifications for the job

rumor: information that has been presented as fact but has not been confirmed

sadness: a state of sorrow and unhappiness

scope of practice: written laws or statutes within each state that define what certified or licensed health care workers can do

selective comprehension: focusing attention toward the part of a conversation that is most interesting during the communication process, while paying little attention to anything else

selective memory: the process in which only certain things are remembered (usually the positive), while other things are forgotten

self-confident attitude: focusing on the positive aspects of oneself to help accomplish goals in a positive manner

self-esteem: personal feeling about oneself

self-motivation: awareness of personal skills and abilities that are then developed to full potential; desire to achieve on your own

service industry: business providing a service to others

sexual abuse: any inappropriate sexual touch or act

short-range goals: goals to be accomplished within 1 month

social space: the distance of 4 to 12 feet from a patient

stress: how the mind and body react to an environment that is largely shaped by perceptions of an event or situation

tact: consideration in interacting with others

telephone etiquette: focusing attention on word choice and quality of voice during telephone conversations to ensure effective communication

territoriality: the process of claiming certain space as one's own

time management: using time and energy in a productive way to help accomplish tasks

trust: consistent behavior that re-ensures the confidence of others, co-workers, and patients

trustworthy attitude: the use of honesty, dependability, and responsibility to gain the trust of others

undirected thinking: a free-flowing thinking process that can include both daydreaming and dreaming while asleep

upward communication: initiated from the staff employees and flows upward to the person or persons in charge

values: a person's beliefs, which are formed through thoughts, feelings, and actions

verbal abuse: occurs when spoken words are meant to hurt another person's self-esteem

verbal communication: the use of spoken words, as in conversations, oral reports, and voice mail, to communicate

vertical communication: a combination of upward and downward communication

vertical thinking: a logical type of thinking that makes step-by-step assumptions based on past experiences

victim attitude: the continual attitude that "everything happens to me" and that one is helpless to change the situation

visualization: to have a mental picture of something

worry: to feel uneasy because of anxiety or troubles

written communication: a form of communication that is written and organized in a precise and thorough manner; can include graphs, films, and reports

INDEX

Page numbers in *italics* indicate figures.

A

Abandonment, 225
Abuse, 220–221
Acceptance, as stage of grief, 222, *222*
Acronyms, 6, *6*, 11–12
Action plans, 58–60
Active euthanasia, 223
Active listening, 141–142, 153
Activity levels, as communication barrier, 137
Advance directives, 230, *231–232*, 235
Against medical advice (AMA), 225
Agendas, 169
All-channel communication, *163*, 164
American Hospital Association, 227, *228–229*
Analogies, 100
Anger, as stage of grief, 222, *222*
Aphasia, 140
Appearance, 120
Assertiveness, 19
Associative thinking, 98, *99*
Attitude
    caring, *22*, 22–23
    as communication barrier, 138, 151
    defined, 20
    negative, 27, 29, 30, 40
    positive, 26–28, 30, 37–38
    professional, 20, 36–37
    self-confident, 19
    trustworthy, 20–21, *21*
    victim, 29
Authority lines, 160, *160*

B

Bad stress, 70–71, *71, 72*, 82
Bargaining, as stage of grief, 222, *222*
Barriers
    to communication, 136–140, *138, 139*, 151–152
    to creative thinking, 100

to listening, 141, 152–153
Battery, 224
Body language, 119–120, 149
Brain death, 223
Brainstorming, 98–100, 107–108, 111–112, 167–168, 174
Brain teaser, 111, *111*
Breathing, for stress management, 81, 86

C

Caffeine, 80, 86
Calendars, 53, *53*, 54, 63–64
Cardiopulmonary resuscitation (CPR), 6
Career/professional goals, 46, 57
Career steps, 197, *198*
Caring attitude, *22*, 22–23
Cell phones, 51
Chain of communication, *163*, 163–164
Change
    defining opportunity for, 96–97, 105–106
    resistance to, 140
    willingness to, 24
Charting, 182–184, *183*, 194
Charts, patient, 177–178, *179*, 191
Chemical restraints, 230
Chief complaint, 178
Classical conditioning, 4
Close-ended questions, 142
Code of ethics, 238–239
Cognitive processes, 90. *See also* Thinking
Cohesiveness, 164
Colleagues, conferring with, 178–179, *179*
Comfort levels, 137
Committees, 174–175
Communication. *See also* Listening
    all channel, *163*, 164
    chain of, *163*, 163–164
    defined, 115
    diagonal, 159
    distortion of, 129–130

Communication (*Continued*)
  downward, 159
  flow of, 159–160
  horizontal, 159
  importance, 127, 150, 170, 190
  nonverbal, 115, 119–121, *121,* 124, 130
  one-way, 128
  with patients, 149, 154
  patterns within groups, *163,* 163–164
  recording and reporting information, 149, *150*
  technological, 147–148
  two-way, 128
  types, 115, 119, 128–129
  upward, 159
  verbal, 115, 122–124, 130–132
  vertical, 159
  web sites for, 148
  wheel of, *163,* 164
  written, 115, 124–127, 132–133
Communication barriers
  environmental, 136–137, *138,* 151
  personal, 137–140, *139,* 151–152
Communication channels, 157–158, 160–161, 171
Communication networks, 157–158, *158*
Communication process, 115–118, *116, 117*
Community goals, 47, 58
Competency, 18, 23–25, *24,* 208
Competitive goals, 162
Complacency, 138
Complaining, 78
Comprehension, selective, 138
Computerized charting, 184
Computers, and time management, 51
Concept maps, 98, *99*
Conferring with colleagues, 178–179, *179*
Confidentiality
  and charting, 183
  medical ethics, 217–218, *219,* 237, 240
  and social space, 185–186
Conformity, 164–165, 173
Constructive concern, 76
Conversations, mirroring, 131
Cooperative goals, 162
Coors (company), 100
Cover letters, 202, *203,* 212
CPR, 6
Creative thinking, 92, 93, 98, 100, 104–105
Creativity, peak periods of, 107
Critical thinking, 5–6, 92, 93, 104
Criticism, constructive, 24–25
Cross-training, 77
Customer relations, 144–145, 146–147, 153

D
Daily to-do lists, 54–55, 64–65
Daydreaming, 141
Death and dying, 221–223, *222,* 237–238
De Bono, Edward, 92
Decision making
  defined, 95

  evaluating impact of, 101, 111
  process, 95–101, *96, 99,* 105–112
Decoding, 116
Deductive reasoning, 91, 103, 104
Denial, as stage of grief, 221, *222*
Dependability, 21, 207
Depression, 74, 222, *222*
Diagonal communication, 159
Difference, making a, 30–31, 189
Directed thinking, 94
Distress, 70–71, *71, 72,* 82
"Do not resuscitate" (DNR) order, 235
Downward communication, 159
Durable power of attorney, 230, *233–234*

E
Educational goals, 46, 58
E-mail, 147–148
Emotional barriers, to communication, 137–138
Empathy, 22, 208
Encoding, 116
Endorphins, 28, 80
Enthusiasm, 25
Enunciation, 123
Environmental barriers
  to communication, 136–137, *138,* 151
  to listening, 141, 152
Ethics, 217. *See also* Medical ethics
Ethics, code of, 238–239
Eustress, 70–71, *71, 72,* 82
Euthanasia, 223, 237–238
Exercise, 80, 85
Extraordinary care, 223
Eye contact, 119, 180

F
Facial expressions, 119
False imprisonment, 224–225
Feedback
  in active listening, 142, 153
  in communication process, 117–118, 122, 124, 129
  in interpersonal relationships, 208–209, 214
Feedback and follow-up stage, of patient encounter, 182–184
Fires, handling, *6*
First impressions, 26, 36, 37, 120, 145
Focused task groups, 164
Formal communication channels, 158
Formal groups, 161
Forms
  medical history, *219*
  study schedule, *9*
Fraud, 227
Functional résumés, 199, *200*

G
Goals
  career/professional, 46, 57
  community, 47, 58
  competitive, 162

cooperative, 162
educational, 46, 58
group, 162
importance, 43
long-range, 47, *48,* 57–60
medium-range, 47, *48,* 60–63
personal, 46, 57–58
refining, 58–60
setting, *44,* 44–45, 47, 57–58, 60–63
short-range, 47, *48,* 60–63
and time management, 50, *50*
types, 46–47
Good stress, 70–71, *71, 72,* 82
Gossip, 160, 161
Gossip Game, 129–130, 172
Grapevine, 158, 160–161
Grief, stages of, 221–222, *222*
Group assessment, 165–166, 172, 173
Group communication patterns, *163,* 163–164
Group dynamics, 162–165
Group goals, 162
Group interaction, 164–165
Groups
formal, 161
informal, 161
social support, 78, 85
Groupthink, 165, 173
Guided imagery, 81, 86

H
Habits, good, 39
Health care professional characteristics, 206–209, 213, 214
Health care proxy, 230, *233–234*
Health Insurance Portability and Accountability Act (HIPAA), 225–226
Hearing, 140, 141. *See also* Listening
Honesty, 21
Horizontal communication, 159
Hospice care, 222, 237–238
Humor, 27–28, 78

I
Ideas
evaluating and selecting, 101, 108–110
generating, 98–100, 106–108
implementing, 101, 110
Idioms, 26
Imagery, visual, 81, 86
Inductive reasoning, 91, 104
Informal communication channels, 158, 160–161
Informal groups, 161
Informed consent, 224
Intentional negligence, 224–227
Interpersonal skills, 208–209
Interviews, 204–206, 213, 214
Intimate space, *187,* 187–188
Introductory stage, of patient encounter, 180–181, 191
Invasion of privacy, 225, 226
"I" statements, 23

J
Job openings, 201–202, 212

K
Kübler-Ross, Elizabeth, 221–222

L
Language, as communication barrier, 139, *139,* 151–152. *See also* Medical terminology
Lateral communication, 159
Lateral thinking, 92, *93*
Lay language, 139, *139. See also* Medical terminology
Leadership, 166–167, 173–174
Learning
enthusiasm for, 24, 25
process, 5–6, 11–12
Legal issues, 224–227, 236
Leisure, 79–80
Lines of authority, 160, *160*
Listening, 140–143, *144. See also* Communication
active, 141–142, 153
barriers to, 141, 152–153
case study, 153
versus hearing, 140
methods, 141–143, *144*
in oral communication, 124
Lists, 54–55, 64–65
Living wills, 230, *231–232,* 235
Logical thinking, 90–91, 103
Long-range goals, 47, *48,* 57–60
Long-term care facilities, 230

M
Malpractice, 227
Malpractice insurance, 239
Medical ethics, 217–223, 237–238
confidentiality, 217–218, *219,* 237, 240
death and dying, 221–223, *222,* 237–238
euthanasia, 223, 237–238
importance, 236
respect, 218, 220, 237
trust, 220–221, 237
Medical history forms, *219*
Medical terminology, 116–117, 118, 123, 139, *139*
exercises, 178, 191–192
Meditation, 81, 86–87
Medium-range goals, 47, *48,* 60–63
Meetings, 168–170
Memory, selective, 138
Memory skills, 6, 11–12
Memos, *127,* 132–133
Mercy killing, 223
Military time, 183–184
Minutes, meeting, 169–170
Mirroring, 131
Mistakes, 24–25
Mixed messages, 130
Mnemonics, 6, 12. *See also* Acronyms
Music, as stress reliever, 78

N

Negative attitude, 27, 29, 30, 40
Negative thinking, 75, 84–85
Negligence, 224–227
Nine dot puzzle, 111, *111*
Noise, as communication barrier, 136
Nonverbal communication, 115, 119–121, *121,* 124, 130
Norms, 162–163, 173
Note taking, 4
Nutrition, 80, 85–86

O

Objectives, 46, 58–60
Olympic training program, 48
One-way communication, 128
Open-ended questions, 142, 153
Oral communication, 115, 122–124, 130–132
Organizational charts, 157, *158,* 171
Outlining, 4–5, 11
Overorganizing, 51
Overplanning, 51
Oz Principle, The (Connors, Smith, and Hickman), 29

P

Parliamentary procedure, 169
Passive euthanasia, 223
Patient assessment, 181–182
Patient Care Partnership, The, 227, *228–229*
Patient education, 149, 154
Patient encounter
    preparing for, 177–179, *179*
    stages, 179–184, 191, 192
Patients
    making a difference to, 189
    respecting space of, 185–188, *186, 187,* 193
    rights, 227, *228–229,* 230
Patient transport, 220
Peak periods, 55
Persistent vegetative state, 223
Personal barriers
    to communication, 137–140, *139,* 151–152
    to listening, 141, 152–153
Personal goals, 46, 57–58
Personal space, 120, 186, *187*
PHI (Protected Health Information), 226
Physical abuse, 220
Physical and mental characteristics, as listening barrier, 141
Physical arrangement, as communication barrier, 137
Physical restraints, 230
Planning, 50–51
Plateau period, 47
Portfolios, xv–xvi
Positive attitude, 26–28, 30, 37–38
Positive thinking, 84–85
Poster presentations, 194, 239
Postinterview stage, 205–206
Practice, scope of, 224, 238
Preconceptions, 141
Preinterview stage, 204
Prejudice, 138, 151

Premises, in logical thinking, 91
Priorities, setting, 51, 52
Privacy, invasion of, 225, 226
Proactive thinking, 91
Procrastination, 51–53
Profession
    health occupations as, 20
    investigating, 214, 238–239
Professional attitude, 20, 36–37
Professional image, 210–211
Progressive muscle relaxation, 81, 87
Project teams, 164
Pronunciation, 123
Protected Health Information (PHI), 226
Protocols, 224
Psychological abuse, 220
Public speaking, 148, 154
Punctuality, 207

Q

Quality, commitment to, 206–207
Questions
    close-ended, 142
    open-ended, 142, 153

R

Reactive thinking, 91
Reasoning. *See also* Thinking
    deductive, 91, 103, 104
    inductive, 91, 104
Reframing, 77, 84–85
Rejuvenation, 78, 85
Relaxation techniques, 80–81, 86–87
Resident's Bill of Rights, 230
Respect, 22, 208, 218, 220, 237
Responsibility, 21
Rest, 79
Restraints, 230
Résumés, 199, *200,* 201, 212
Right to die issues, 223, 230, *231–234,* 235
Roles, individual, 162–163
Rumor, 160

S

Sadness, 74
Safety issues, 239
Scope of practice, 224, 238
Selective comprehension, 138
Selective memory, 138
Self-absorption, 141
Self-assessment
    assertiveness, 19
    caring attitude, 23
    competent attitude, 25
    health care practitioner characteristics, 209
    job suitability, 198–199, 212
    leadership skills, 167
    listening, 143
    stress management, 72
    stress signals, 75
    time management, 49

trustworthy attitude, 21
  verbal communication, 131–132
Self-care, 7, 12–13
Self-confident attitude, 19
Self-esteem, *17,* 17–18
Self-fulfilling prophecy, 30, 75
Self-motivation, 16, 35
Self-talk, 30, 38, 75, 84–85
Serotonin, 80
Service industry, health occupations as, 20
Sexual abuse, 181, 220–221
Seyle, Hans, 70
Short-range goals, 47, *48,* 60–63
Sincerity, 22
Sleep, 79
SOAPIE notes, 192–193
Social space, 185–186, *186*
Social support groups, 78, 85
Sprain treatment, 11
Standard English, 131
Stress, *69*
  bad, 70–71, *71, 72,* 82
  defined, 69
  good, 70–71, *71, 72,* 82
  producers, *72,* 75, 77, 83
  signals, *74,* 74–75, 84, 87
  types, 70–71, *71,* 82
Stress management, 67–88
  emotional strategies, 76–78, *79*
  importance, 68
  overview, 73, *73*
  physical strategies, 79–81
  and time management, 77–78
  tips, *81*
  worry, 73, 76, 84
Stretching, 80
Study skills, 2–14
  action plans, 10, *10,* 12–13
  daily preparation, 3
  good study habits, 4–5, 11
  learning and testing process, 5–6, 11–12
  self-care, 7, 12–13
  study schedule, *8,* 9, *9*
  time and place for study, 4, 10
Subconscious, 107
Success
  attributes, 32
  characteristics, 15–41
  definitions, 16, 33

T
Tact, 23
Technological barriers, to communication, 137
Technological communication, 147–148
Telephone etiquette, 145–146, *146,* 154
Telephones, and time management, 51
Terminally ill patients, 77, 221–222, *222*
Territoriality, 185, 188
Test-taking strategies, 6
Thinking
  associative, 98, *99*

  creative, 92, 93, 98, 100, 104–105
  critical, 5–6, 92, 93, 104
  deductive, 91, 103, 104
  directed, 94
  inductive, 91, 104
  lateral, 92, *93*
  logical, 90–91, 103
  negative, 75, 84–85
  positive, 84–85
  proactive, 91
  reactive, 91
  reframing, 77, 84–85
  undirected, 94
  vertical, 92, *93*
Time and distance, as communication barrier, 137
Time management
  benefits, 43
  and goals, 50, *50*
  importance, 49, 56, 102
  and stress management, 77–78
  techniques, 50–55
Time wasters, 50–53, 63
Touch, 120
Treating and monitoring stage, of patient encounter, 182
Trust, 208, 220–221, 237
Trustworthy attitude, 20–21, *21*
Two-way communication, 128

U
Undirected thinking, 94
Unintentional negligence, 224, 227
Universal precautions, 193
Upward communication, 159

V
Vacation, 78
Values, 18, *18,* 20, 34–35
Vegetative state, 223
Velcro, invention of, 100
Verbal abuse, 220
Verbal communication, 115, 122–124, 130–132
Vertical communication, 159
Vertical thinking, 92, *93*
Victim attitude, 29
Visual imagery, 81, 86
Visualization, 47, 98, *99*
Voice, manner and tone of, 122–123, 130–131

W
Warming up, before exercise, 80
Water, drinking, 80, 85
Web sites, 148
Wheel of communication, *163,* 164
Worry, 51, 52–53, 73, 76, 84
Written communication, 115, 124–127, 132–133

Y
Yoga breathing, 81, 86
"You" statements, 23